Five Pillars of Brain Fitness

Five Pillars of Brain Fitness

A User's Manual for Lifelong Brain Fitness

Meredith Patterson RN,BSN and Pete Goodwin

Contents

Acknowledgments

T HE AUTHORS WISH to thank the many nurses, doctors, and research professionals who so generously shared their knowledge about the etiology and progression of dementing diseases.

We especially thank the family and professional caregivers who shared their stories about caring for a loved one suffering with dementia.

Preface

You start to notice it happening more often. What was the name of that movie we saw last week? You know, the one with that actor married to that attractive actress with the big lips? You walk into the garage and stand there for a minute or two wondering why you went in there. And for the second time this week you can't find your car keys or the TV remote. You struggle for several long moments trying to remember the name of a fellow churchgoer you've known for many years.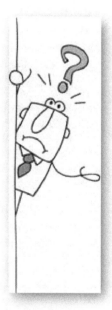

You experience a wave of anxiety as you recall that you're about the same age as your mother was when she first started forgetting things. With trepidation, you ask yourself, "Why is Mom going backward?" as she succumbs, inexorably, to the damage to the brain caused by Alzheimer's disease.

You try to put the fear to rest by reassuring yourself that this is all just a natural part of aging. After all, many of your friends report the same experiences. But in the back of your mind, you worry that you will inevitably follow the same path as your mother.

Like many people, you think that the likelihood of developing Alzheimer's disease is mostly determined by your genetic makeup, that there's nothing much you can do about it, and that you'll just have to wait for that magic-bullet cure and hope it comes in time to save you.

If you find yourself nodding in agreement, then you may be surprised to learn that genetics is not the sole determiner of Alzheimer's disease and that there are indeed several strategies you can employ to significantly reduce your risk of developing Alzheimer's. That's why we wrote this book.

We worked in the world of Alzheimer's and senior care for many years. When admitting a new resident to one of the dementia care assisted-living facilities at which we worked, we would inevitably be asked the same question by the adult children of the new resident: "Is there anything I can do so I don't end up like my mother or father? Can I do something to help prevent losing my memory?"

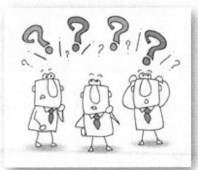

As it turns out, there is, according to research published by Deborah Barnes, PhD, assistant adjunct professor of psychiatry, and Kristine Yaffe, MD, professor of psychiatry, neurology, and epidemiology, both at the University of California, San Francisco.[1] They found that seven common modifiable factors are associated with lowering the risk of developing Alzheimer's: quitting smoking, increasing physical activity, enhancing mental activity, controlling blood pressure and diabetes, and managing obesity and depression.

Based on these researchers' findings and the research of many other neuroscientists and physicians, we have developed a program that we call the *Five Pillars of Brain Fitness*. The program looks at the five lifestyle factors most likely to influence the health and fitness of your brain, with the goal of improving memory and cognitive ability and significantly reducing your risk of developing Alzheimer's disease or delaying the onset and slowing the progression of the disease. As an added bonus, following the *Five Pillars of Brain Fitness* guidelines also contributes to lowering your risk of cardiovascular and pulmonary disease, as well as diabetes. Physical and mental exercises, proper nutrition, staying socially active, and managing stress are the foundations of the *Five Pillars of Brain Fitness* program. As with any fitness program,

1 Deborah E. Barnes and Kristine Yaffe, "The Projected Effect of Risk Factor Reduction on Alzheimer's Disease Prevalence," *The Lancet Neurology* 10, no. 9 (2011): 819–28, doi:10.1016/S1474-4422(11)70072-2.

discipline, consistency, and a willingness to learn new techniques are key to success.

We're often asked, "At what age is it best to start my brain fitness training?" The answer is at any age. From the time you are born on into your senior years, following the *Five Pillars of Brain Fitness* guidelines will help your brain grow and thrive. It's never too late to start.

It helps to have the support of family and friends to achieve success. Recruit a partner so that you can each encourage and support each other in achieving your goals. Perhaps your spouse, children, or siblings or a close friend can work with you as you implement your brain fitness program. Each of us is different, and each of us has areas of strength and weakness. Focus on maximizing your strengths and improving your weaknesses.

If your goal is to lose weight and you sign up for a diet program but only follow it one day a month, you're not likely to see much progress. Similarly, if your goal is physical fitness and you join a gym but only work out once a month, you're unlikely to see much improvement. So it is with achieving maximum brain fitness. If you only follow the five pillars one day a month, don't expect to see much change. You don't have to follow the five pillars perfectly every day to gain some benefit, but following them at least three to four days a week is recommended.

A paper published by a Duke University researcher in 2006 found that more than 40 percent of the actions people performed each day weren't due to decision making but to habits.[2] Good habits can be difficult to adopt, and bad habits can be difficult to eliminate, but as Charles Duhigg reports in his book *The Power of Habit*, "Habits aren't destiny...we can transform our businesses, our communities, and our lives." So make following the *Five Pillars of Brain Fitness* a habit in your life. Build a better brain, sharpen your memory, improve your cognitive skills, and significantly reduce your risk of developing Alzheimer's as you age by following the *Five Pillars of Brain Fitness* program.

---

2 Charles Duhigg, *The Power of Habit* (New York: Random House, 2012), xvi.

Introduction

The Senior Tsunami

ON JANUARY 1, 2011, the United States reached a demographic milestone. The first members of the post–World War II baby boomer generation (individuals born between 1946 and 1964) began to turn sixty-five. Since that day, and for the following eighteen years, more than ten thousand people a day reach their sixty-fifth birthdays.[3] According to Pew Research Center population projections for 2030, when all of the baby boomers have turned sixty-five, fully 18 percent of the US population will be that age or older. Our country is aging for other reasons as well. Breakthroughs in medical technology and pharmacology are extending lives. Our nation's birthrate also continues to decline, meaning that there are fewer young people as a percentage of our population. The National Center for Health Statistics at the Centers for Disease Control and Prevention states that the 2012 birthrate was the lowest rate in the seventy-three years the government has been collecting the data.[4] The decline was across all racial and ethnic groups.

While extending life span is an exciting prospect, increasing age also poses a concern for our health and fitness. Few want to lead a long life if they are afflicted with disease, frailty, or dementia. When surveyed, working-age individuals cite finances as their biggest worry, but an AARP study of

3 "Baby Boomers Retire," Pew Research Center, December 29, 2010, http://www.pewresearch.org/daily-number/baby-boomers-retire/.

4 Joyce A. Martin et al., "Births: Final Data for 2013," National Vital Statistics Reports, January 15, 2015,
http://www.cdc.gov/nchs/data/nvsr/nvsr64/nvsr64_01.pdf.

individuals over age fifty revealed health concerns as the number one worry of aging Americans.

The Rising Specter of Alzheimer's Disease

The Centers for Disease Control and Prevention lists the top ten causes of death in the United States as:

1. Heart disease
2. Cancer
3. Chronic lower respiratory disease
4. Stroke
5. Accidents
6. Alzheimer's disease
7. Diabetes
8. Influenza and pneumonia
9. Kidney disease
10. Suicide

Interestingly, even though Alzheimer's disease ranks sixth on the list, when surveyed, seniors cite losing their memory and cognitive abilities among their greatest concerns.

Currently, there are more than five million individuals in the United States afflicted with Alzheimer's disease. Sadly, that number is increasing fast. By 2020, there will be about seven million Americans afflicted, and by 2050 that number is expected to exceed fifteen million.

What It Takes to Succeed

Brainstorm Mind Fitness has a philosophy about brain fitness:

- Brain health practice is supported by consistent, evidence-based research.
- Good brain health is not expensive, nor difficult to achieve, and it is easily practiced in everyday life.

- Brain health is not attributed to one practice but to several lifestyle changes.
- Consistency and willingness to learn are key characteristics to succeed.
- Brain health habits may significantly decrease your risk of having dementia, as well as prevent or delay the onset of symptoms.

In the coming chapters, we lead you through the *Five Pillars of Brain Fitness* one by one, explaining what each pillar is and why it benefits the brain. It's important to remember that brain health is not attributed to one practice but to several lifestyle changes. To be successful, you must work on each of the five pillars. Success cannot be achieved by focusing only on one or two of the pillars. Remember, also, that consistency and willingness to learn are key characteristics for success. Set goals for each of the five pillars and track the results weekly.

See appendix 7 for a sample progress chart.

Just as you can improve your physical fitness by working on diet and exercise, so you can improve your brain fitness by focusing on the *Five Pillars of Brain Fitness*.

Dementia: The Journey Back to Childhood

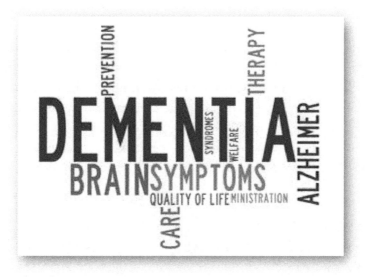

Have you ever had any of these experiences?

- Misplaced your car keys
- Misplaced the TV remote control
- Misplaced your eyeglasses
- Walked into a room and couldn't remember why
- Opened the refrigerator door and couldn't remember what you wanted
- Couldn't remember the name of a famous actor/actress
- Couldn't remember the title of a book or movie
- Couldn't remember the name of someone you've met several times
- Forgot to go to an appointment

Most of us have had experiences similar to these and, when we do, we inevitably feel that wave of anxiety sweep over us wondering if this is a harbinger of emerging Alzheimer's disease.

Well, you can relax. All of those experiences are examples of normal age-related forgetfulness. Occasional memory lapses, such as forgetting why you walked into a room or having difficulty recalling a person's name, become more common as we approach our fifties and sixties. It's comforting to know that this minor forgetfulness is a normal sign of aging and not a sign of dementia.

But other types of memory loss, such as forgetting appointments or becoming momentarily disoriented in a familiar place, may indicate mild cognitive impairment (MCI), a more serious form of memory impairment, People with MCI often find themselves disoriented in time and place and unable to name common objects or recognize once-familiar people. More serious problems with memory and cognition are signs of dementia.

Many people ask us, "What's the distinction between dementia and Alzheimer's disease?" Let's clear that up first.

Dementia Defined

The term *dementia* comes from Latin, originally meaning "madness," from *de* "without" + *ment*, "mind." In medicine, dementia refers to a set of symptoms, such as memory loss, confusion with time and place, cognitive impairment, irrational thoughts, irrational feelings, problems with planning, problems finding words, problems understanding what others are 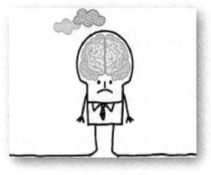 saying, and, eventually, problems with balance and movement.

Technically, dementia is not a diagnosis; instead, it is a set of symptoms caused by an underlying malady. The symptoms of dementia indicate that something is going on in the brain that is causing the brain to malfunction. A medical practitioner needs to determine what is causing a patient's symptoms of dementia in order to arrive at a diagnosis. The symptoms of dementia can be related to several different conditions. Some causes of dementia are treatable, such as:

- Blood clots in the brain
- Normal pressure hydrocephalous
- Brain tumors
- Lyme's disease
- Hypo- or hyperthyroidism
- Hypoglycemia (low blood sugar)
- Vitamin B12 deficiency
- Chronic liver failure
- Chronic renal failure

Other diseases that cause the symptoms of dementia are progressive, incurable, and ultimately fatal. These include:

- Alzheimer's disease
- Vascular dementia (damage to the blood vessels in the brain)
- Dementia with Lewy bodies
- Parkinson's disease
- Frontotemporal dementia
- Creutzfeldt-Jakob disease (mad cow disease)
- Huntington's disease

What Causes Alzheimer's Disease?

By far, Alzheimer's disease is the most common cause of dementia. It is estimated that 60–80 percent of dementia cases are the result of Alzheimer's disease.[5] Like all types of dementia, Alzheimer's is caused by brain cell damage and death. When researchers examine brain tissue from people who die from

---

5 "Types of Dementia," Alzheimer's Association, 2016, http://www.alz.org/dementia/types-of-dementia.asp.

Alzheimer's disease, they find two common causes of brain cell death. First, in the spaces between neurons, there exist clumps of tissue called *beta amyloid plaques*.[6] These plaque formations cause nearby neurons to become inflamed and eventually die.

Second, within the neurons, researchers see what are called *neurofibrillary tangles* (NFTs).[7] These are damaged and tangled microtubules that, in a healthy brain, aid in communicating signals along the neuron. NFTs are caused by decomposition of tau proteins within the neuron. NFTs cause brain cells to malfunction and eventually die.

As yet, researchers don't know what causes the two proteins to malfunction and damage brain tissue. There have been hundreds of clinical trials to try and understand the pathology of Alzheimer's disease.

The Role of Heredity

Many people worry that they may be at risk for developing Alzheimer's disease as they age, especially if they have had a parent or grandparent who suffered from the disease. Heredity does seem to play some role in increasing the risk of developing Alzheimer's. Individuals with a family history of Alzheimer's are somewhat more likely to develop the disease than those with no family history. Individuals whose mothers had Alzheimer's appear to be more at risk than those whose fathers had the disease.[8]

There is a rare form of genetically based Alzheimer's disease that strikes younger adults, sometimes as young as thirty-five, and progresses rapidly. It is called *early-onset familial Alzheimer's disease*. Fortunately, this disease

6 "More about Plaques," Alzheimer's Association, 2011, https://www.alz.org/braintour/plaques.asp.

7 "More about Tangles," Alzheimer's Association, 2011, https://www.alz.org/braintour/tangles.asp.

8 Robyn A. Honea et al., "Maternal Family History Is Associated with Alzheimer's Disease Biomarkers," *Journal of Alzheimer's Disease* 31, no. 3 (2012): 659–68, doi:10.3233/JAD-2012-120676.

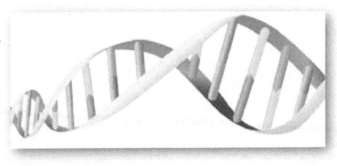

accounts for fewer than 4 percent of existing Alzheimer's cases.[9] By far, most Alzheimer's cases occur in individuals over age sixty-five. Approximately 5 percent of adults sixty-five years of age and older have Alzheimer's, and almost 40 percent of those eighty-five years and older have the disease.[10]

But a family history of the disease does not guarantee you'll develop Alzheimer's. Even if you have a family history of Alzheimer's, following the *Five Pillars of Brain Fitness* can reduce your risk of developing the disease.

Preventable Causes

As noted in the preface, researchers Deborah Barnes and Kristine Yaffe determined that about half of all cases of Alzheimer's disease result from seven preventable causes (diabetes, midlife hypertension, midlife obesity, smoking, depression, cognitive inactivity, and physical inactivity).[11] Their research found that a 25 percent reduction in all seven factors could potentially prevent between one and three million cases of Alzheimer's disease per year worldwide.

These findings and our own professional insights led us to develop the *Five Pillars of Brain Fitness* program, designed to help aging adults keep their memories intact and their cognitive capabilities sharp and, most importantly, significantly reduce their risk of developing Alzheimer's disease.

9 Thomas D. Bird, "Early-Onset Familial Alzheimer Disease," National Center for Biotechnical Information, Last Revision October 18, 2012, http://www.ncbi.nlm.nih.gov/books/NBK1236/.

10 Alzheimer's Association, "2015 Alzheimer's Disease Facts and Figures," *Alzheimer's & Dementia* 11, no. 3 (2015): 332–416.

11

Five Pillars of Brain Fitness Overview

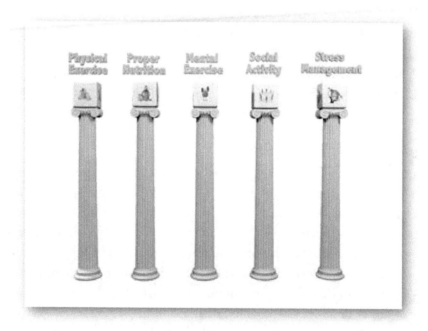

AS NOTED EARLIER, we have distilled the findings of Deborah Barnes and Kristine Yaffe, along with many other researchers, into five key "pillars" of brain fitness that can make the biggest difference in maximizing brain fitness and minimizing the risk of developing Alzheimer's disease. Each pillar represents a lifestyle activity that, if concentrated on, can make noticeable and significant differences in your brain's fitness. Here are the five pillars:

1. Physical Exercise
2. Proper Nutrition

3. Mental Exercises
4. Social Activity
5. Stress Management

Researchers have identified each of these areas as crucial to optimal brain fitness. In the coming chapters, you will learn the science behind each pillar of brain fitness and develop personal goals and a plan for achievement in each area. Sample exercises, worksheets, and measurement tools are provided.

By following the *Five Pillars of Brain Fitness,* you will build a better brain, sharpen your memory, improve your cognitive skills, and significantly reduce your risk of developing Alzheimer's as you age. Let's get started.

Pillar 1: Physical Exercise

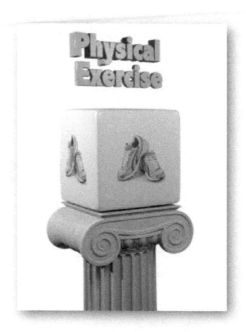

WHAT IF WE told you there was a magic brain pill that has passed hundreds of research studies with flying colors? That it was very inexpensive or often free? That when taken as prescribed might cut your risk of having dementia *in half*? And that the "side effects" of such a pill included lowering your blood pressure, keeping your weight down, and making you generally more energetic throughout your day?

Of course you would want this magic pill, and we would all desperately wish this fairy tale to come true. Only the benefits we've described don't come by swallowing a pill or a potion—but they do come with regular physical exercise.

If you're a person who has never been convinced that exercise should be at the top of your priority list, please reconsider. Quite simply, it is the single most important lifestyle factor that underlies brain health, period.

In this chapter, we'll look at how exercise alters brain chemistry—making the brain more resilient, better nourished, and quicker to soak up information. Then we'll delve into research studies on just what type of and how much exercise is needed for benefits. Finally, we'll make a few suggestions to kick-start your own brain-training program.

Oxygenation

The most obvious effect of exercise is that it makes you breathe harder, right? When you're climbing a flight of stairs or cranking out the miles on a treadmill, your heart is pumping faster and more oxygen is being carried by your red blood cells to all the places that oxygen is needed in the body—and primarily to the brain.

That's right! The brain is an oxygen-hungry organ and consumes 20–25 percent of the body's oxygen demands.[12] The brain needs nourishment—in the form of food for fuel and air for oxygen—and it requires it constantly. Most people know that "brain death" can happen in just a few minutes if deprived of oxygen.

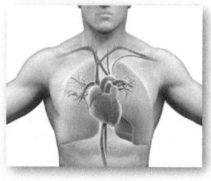

But even more interesting is where the oxygen travels in the brain regions; specifically, you'll see the heaviest cerebral blood flow volume in the region called the *dentate gyrus*, housed within the hippocampus. This is the part of the brain that is crucial for memory and learning. More and more, research points to aerobic exercise as essential to working memory, planning, and organization— all aspects of the higher level thinking we call *executive control*.[13]

In addition to improving oxygenation, increased blood flow also provides the brain with more glucose (blood sugar), the fuel that powers the brain.

The Magic Molecule: BDNF

We can all agree that good blood flow is essential for the brain to hum along smoothly and efficiently. But another chemistry shift happens with

---

12 "Cerebral Blood Flow and Oxygen Consumption," CNS Clinic, 2016, http://www.humanneurophysiology.com/cbfo2consumption.htm.

13 Charles H. Hillman, Kirk I. Erickson, and Arthur F. Kramer, "Be Smart, Exercise Your Heart: Exercise Effects on Brain and Cognition," *Nature Reviews Neuroscience* 9, no. 1 (2008): 58–65, doi:10.1038/nrn2298.

exercise—namely, the production of a molecule called *brain-derived ueurotrophic factor*, or BDNF.

What is BDNF? Discovered in 1990, BDNF is a naturally occurring molecule that helps to solidify neuronal connections, improving the signal strength of synapses and generally supporting neuron growth. Dr. John Ratey, author of *Spark: The Revolutionary New Science of Exercise and the Brain*, describes BDNF as "Miracle Gro for the brain."[14]

The subject of many studies, BDNF is enhanced naturally by many things—and most readily by physical exercise. When BDNF is elevated, the brain is primed for new learning. For example, one study examined the ability of participants to learn new vocabulary words. Their speed in such a task improved by 20 percent after exercising.[15]

Increasing oxygenation and abundant BDNF molecules are huge bonus benefits of a physical exercise workout; by now, you are likely looking at your gym time in a whole new light. No longer are you huffing and puffing just to look good in a bathing suit (although that's definitely nice), but your brain will operate better as well.

Spurred on by an abundance of BNDF and oxygen, we can conclude that exercise benefits the ability to learn in three specific ways:

1). It optimizes the mind- set to improve alertness, motivation, and attention.;
2. It prepares and encourages brain cells to bind to one another, increasing connectivity.
3. It spurs the development of new nerve cells from stem cells in the hippocampus.

---

14 John J. Ratey, with Eric Hagerman, *Spark: The Revolutionary New Science of Exercise and the Brain* (New York: Little, Brown, 2008), 19.

15 Bernward Winter et al., "High Impact Running Improves Learning," *Neurobiology of Learning and Memory* 87, no. 4 (2007): 597–609, doi:10.1016/j.nlm.2006.11.003.

Exercise as a Means to Prevent Brain Shrinkage

One thing we know without a doubt is that size matters, at least as far as the brain is concerned. A healthy brain is one that is well fed, robust, and densely populated with neurons. Shrinkage or atrophy of the brain, especially in areas critical for new learning, is never a good thing.

The problem is that, with age, the brain has a natural trajectory of shrinkage beginning somewhere in the sixth decade of life. This takes place even in the absence of neurocognitive diseases, such as dementia. Of particular concern is the shrinkage noted in the hippocampus, that part of the brain often referred to as the seat of new learning.

But research shows us that shrinkage can be prevented—effectively setting back the clock—simply through exercise. One study that looked at this aspect of brain aging, and its reversal, published its findings online in *Proceedings of the National Academy of Sciences*. The research team found that adults aged fifty-five to eighty who walked around a track for forty minutes, three days a week for a year, increased the volume of their hippocampi, the brain region that is involved in memory, learning, and spatial reasoning. Older adults assigned to a stretching routine showed no hippocampal growth.

The 120 previously sedentary older adults recruited for the study did not yet have diagnosable dementia but were experiencing typical age-related reduction of the hippocampus, according to study MRIs. In other words, they were starting to have those "senior moments" that we think of as inevitable.

The growth of the hippocampus increased 2.12 percent in the left hippocampus and 1.97 percent in the right hippocampus, which sounds modest, but it effectively turned back the clock by one to two years. The stretching group, on the other hand, experienced continued reduction in pace with expected age-related losses, losing on average 1.40 percent and 1.43 percent in the volume of their left and right hippocampi, respectively. Subjects in both the walking and stretching groups

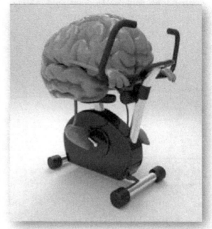

improved in accuracy when tested on a spatial memory test. But those who were in better shape—and thus also tended to have larger hippocampi—at the start of the study did the best on the memory tests, suggesting that greater hippocampal volume translates to better memory.

One other measurable benefit came out of this study. Remember the molecule BDNF? The aerobic exercise group also showed higher levels of brain-derived neurotrophic factor.

Can Exercise Help if Memory Is Already Impaired?

It used to be believed that once memory loss became problematic—and diagnosed as mild cognitive impairment or Alzheimer's—that there was no stopping the inevitable slide of further mental decline. But research from the University of Maryland School of Public Health shows that exercise may improve cognitive function in those at risk for Alzheimer's by improving memory efficiency. While some memory loss is normal and to be expected as we age, a diagnosis of *mild cognitive impairment,* or MCI, signals more substantial memory loss and a greater risk for Alzheimer's, for which there currently is no cure.

A study led by Dr. J. Carson Smith, assistant professor in the Department of Kinesiology, was the first to show that an exercise intervention with older adults with MCI (average age of seventy-eight) improved not only memory recall but also brain function, as measured by functional neuroimaging. The findings were published in the *Journal of Alzheimer's Disease.*

Two groups of physically inactive older adults (ranging from sixty to eighty-eight years old) were put on a twelve-week exercise program that focused on regular treadmill walking guided by a personal trainer. By the end of the intervention, both groups, one that included adults with MCI and the other with healthy brain function, improved their cardiovascular fitness by about 10 percent. But improvement didn't stop with physical fitness. Both groups also improved their memory performance and showed enhanced neural efficiency while engaged in memory retrieval tasks. All of this was achieved with a "moderate intensity pace" (activity that increases your heart and makes you sweat but still allows you to have a conversation while doing it). Weekly exercise averaged a total of 150 minutes.

One of the memory tests involved a common memory problem—remembering names. Study participants were asked to identify famous names, and their brain activation was measured while engaged in correctly recognizing a name (e.g., Frank Sinatra or other celebrities well known to adults born in the 1930s and 1940s). In this way, the brain-level activity could be observed when taxed to remember. Tests and imaging were performed both before and after the twelve-week exercise intervention. Brain scans taken after the exercise intervention showed a significant increase in the intensity of brain activation in eleven brain regions as participants correctly identified famous names. The brain regions with improved efficiency corresponded to those involved in the pathology of Alzheimer's disease.

The exercise intervention was also effective in improving word recall via a "list-learning task"—people were read a list of fifteen words and asked to remember and repeat as many words as possible on five consecutive attempts and again after a distraction of being given another list of words.[16]

Exercise as a Modulator to Stress

Anyone who has incorporated regular exercise into their schedules will tell you that, although the program may have been intended for physical improvement, what brings them back to the gym may in fact be the mental "relief" that comes with a good workout. Indeed, exercise is a well-known remedy for stress symptoms, such as depression and anxiety, and, in some countries, is used as a first-line treatment for these disorders.

Although your problems don't magically melt away while you're pounding the treadmill, your ability to deal with those problems rebounds through exercise. In other words, exercise has a way of making the brain more resilient to stress and helps to reverse the damages caused by chronic stress (see Pillar 5: Stress Management).

---

16 Sherrie Bourg Carter, "Has Sleep and Stress Become a Vicious Cycle in Your Life? Why Sleep Should Be on the Top of Your To-Do List," *Psychology Today*, May 27, 2011, https://www.psychologytoday.com/blog/high-octane-women/201105/has-sleep-and-stress-become-vicious-cycle-in-your-life.

The way exercise works to suppress the stress response lies in your brain's ability to alter its chemistry with activity. The physical stress of an elevated heart rate diverts blood flow from the prefrontal cortex to the extremities so suddenly that it's impossible to attend to all those problems you've been ruminating about. Very simply, exercise breaks up the brain's stress feedback loop of worrying, rinse, repeat.

Important hormone changes occur during exercise as well. When stress hormones attack, the body needs the counterbalancing hormone norepinephrine to quiet everything down and modulate the stress response. Think of norepinephrine as your "chill" switch in the face of stress. The act of exercising increases norepinephrine levels, flipping that chill switch on more quickly and returning the brain to a calmer, more rational state.

Other helpful neurotransmitters, such as GABA (gamma aminobutyric Aacid), serotonin, and tryptophan, are enhanced by the exercise effect. GABA is known as the brain's major inhibitor; when you take a prescription antianxiety medication like a benzodiazepine, it binds with GABA receptors. Serotonin is known as the neurotransmitter underlying mood and a sense of well-being. Serotonin and 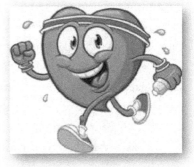 its precursor, tryptophan, are involved in regulating mood and depressive disorders. Physical exercise promotes the production of GABA, serotonin, and tryptophan.

"Stressing" the body through physical exercise has another psychological component as well. Successful workouts lead to a normal state of arousal. In other words, it teaches you to attain a different outcome to arousal—a positive outcome. When the body calms itself after exercise, resuming its usual resting heart rate and blood pressure, the mind tends to follow suit, and you'll find yourself less inclined to worry so much.

Exercise and Depression

As with anxiety and stress, exercise is a powerful antidote to depression, which is a common occurrence in the population. The World Health Organization cites depression as a leading cause of disability in both the United States and Canada. More than ten million Americans take prescription antidepressants.

Key brain chemistry affecting depression includes norepinephrine and serotonin, and it's no surprise that antidepressants target these specific neurotransmitters. Exercise, however, efficiently regulates norepinephrine and serotonin. Dopamine, another neurotransmitter helpful for mood and attention, is also boosted by exercise.

Would exercise be a possible effective substitute for prescription antidepressants? Research suggests so. A landmark study from Duke University in 1999 made a strong case for using exercise in lieu of prescription antidepressants. In this study, 156 participants suffering from depression were divided into three groups: one taking Zoloft, one assigned to a walking exercise program, and one assigned to a jogging exercise program. The exercise groups did thirty minutes of activity three times a week. At the end of sixteen weeks, all three groups had experienced a decrease in depression.

But the interesting thing about this study was the measurement of depression relapse rate six months after the study was concluded. In the exercise groups, the relapse rate was only 8 percent compared to a 38 percent relapse rate in the group taking medication alone. The researchers' conclusion: exercise works better than medication for long-term management of depression.

What Kind of Exercise Is Best, and How Much Should I Do?

If you're like most people, you've read through this chapter wondering when we'd get to the hard part—implementing an exercise program that will work best for brain health while keeping it realistic for all fitness levels. Let's start with some key principals:

1. In order for an exercise program to work, you must choose activities that you will do. It may sound obvious, but if you're told that the best thing in the world for you is to swing kettlebell weights, and you absolutely detest kettlebells ever since you dropped one on your foot, then it's unlikely that you will be lifting any kettlebell weights. There

are several ways to get fit, but only you can do the work, so choose something that suits you.

2. Consistency is the key. Walking once a month won't cut it. We recommend at least three days a week, preferably four, for a minimum of thirty minutes of activity.

3. Make it a priority. Again, this *is* the magic pill, but it's not something you can delegate to an assistant. Consider this: make a plan, and find the time. Get up earlier, go to the gym instead of going to lunch, or exercise before you allow yourself to eat dinner. Do whatever it takes to make exercise your first priority.

4. Start small and set realistic goals; more about this later.

Now to the business of exercise type, duration, and intensity—and what the research tells us.

Aerobic Exercise

Aerobic exercise is what gets the heart pumping, the blood flowing, and the oxygen delivered. Logically, aerobic exercise should be the backbone of most exercise programs for purposes of physical and mental conditioning. Let's summarize again what aerobic exercise does in terms of brain health:

- Increased efficiency of oxygen-carrying ability pumped by the heart and lungs to the body and brain.
- The initiation of the cascade effects of BDNF, serotonin, and other beneficial neurotransmitters and hormones.
- The acceleration of metabolism and fat-burning capacity, resulting in more efficient utilization of insulin.

But more to the point, the effects of aerobic activity are quickly achieved! In a 2007 study conducted by the University of Michigan, when muscle biopsies were compared before and after exercise, researchers concluded that even a single session of exercise completely reversed insulin resistance (a cell's inability to process glucose) the next day.

Intrigued? Let's go a step farther—and faster. What if you mixed regular aerobic activity with higher intensity spurts of exercise, known as *interval training* or *high-impact interval training*? What happens when, for short intervals, the intensity of exercise increases to boost the heart rate to 75–90 percent of its maximum rate? At this speed, aerobic exercise turns anaerobic (literally meaning "without air"), and suddenly you are struggling to breathe and your legs feel rubbery. All of this is due to the muscles entering a state of hypoxia, burning creatine and glycogen and creating 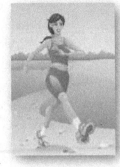 lactic acid. If you've every pushed yourself up a hill by foot or on a bike, you know exactly what we're talking about.

The point of all this agony is that pushing yourself even a little can have profound effects on your brain. In a study from the University of Muenster, Germany, two groups of participants tackled a forty-minute treadmill run. One group stayed at a low-intensity speed while another interspersed sprints of two- to three-minute durations throughout the workout. The results? Compared with the low-intensity group, the sprinters had higher levels of BDNF and improved vocabulary test results by 20 percent.[17]

Before you lace up your running shoes, here are a few tips to save yourself from injury and discouragement. Build an aerobic base gradually, going for a mild elevation in heart rate over a given period of time. Your goal is to build up to thirty minutes of aerobic exercise spread out over a minimum of three to four days a week. Then start your interval spurts after you've established that baseline. If you have other medical considerations, check with your doctor first.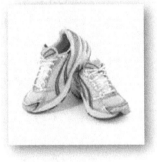

You don't have to be terribly scientific or invest in a lot of techie devices to achieve your fitness level. Measuring your pulse is one way, but you can also use *perceived exertion*. Perceived exertion is whether the exercise feels

---

17 Gayatri Devi, *A Calm Brain: Unlocking Your Natural Relaxation System* (New York: Penguin, 2012), 45–7.

comfortable or difficult at certain speeds; a comfortable low-intensity rate of exercise allows you to talk easily with a companion while exercising.

Strength and Balance Training

Although aerobic exercise is arguably the most direct conduit to brain fitness, strength and balance exercises are also beneficial. Much of the research on nonaerobic exercise focuses on mood and anxiety benefits rather than on learning and memory.

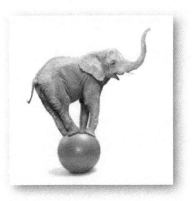

Balance training benefits the cerebellum, the part of the brain that governs balance, coordination, and motor activity sequencing. Known as "the little brain," the cerebellum houses roughly half of all the neurons in your head. Including alternate exercises such as dancing, Pilates, tai chi, and yoga—or anything else that challenges motor coordination and balance—should also be part of your exercise (and brain exercise) program. Zumba dancing counts too!

But I Don't Like to Exercise

Part of a natural distaste for exercising might be built into your genetic disposition, another thing you can blame on your parents. If this is the case, you may require a longer time to get over the hump before exercise becomes a habit. And you're not alone. More than half of all people who begin an exercise program drop out by the time six months have elapsed.

Research points to the fact that consistency of exercise is essential for neural stimulation. At a study conducted by the University of California at Irvine, the BDNF levels of rats were compared to their exercise schedules. Half of the rats ran daily on a treadmill while the other half ran every other day. After three months, the rats that ran daily accelerated their BDNF production more rapidly than the alternate days

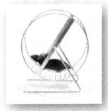

group (150 percent vs. 124 percent after two weeks). Interestingly, it took only two weeks for BDNF levels to flatten without exercise. When the rats returned to running, BDNF levels shot back up in just two days for both groups. The researchers concluded that, although it may be ideal to exercise every day, even intermittent exercise works wonders.

Sticking To It

Like anything else, an exercise program, especially for a neophyte, requires planning and realistic goal setting before implementation. Here are a few tips to keep you on track:

- Walk before you run. Start slow and easy.
- Do whatever type of exercise suits you. When you've reached your fitness plateau, challenge yourself by different or more intense workouts.
- Build your exercise time into your schedule. Make exercise a priority, and let your friends and family know what you will be doing—and, more importantly, why.
- Invite a buddy to exercise with you; this makes both of you accountable to each other.
- Make goals reasonable and specific.
- Exercise in time increments, gradually increasing aerobic activity to thirty minutes in duration.
- Change your routine to keep it interesting.

One More Thing

Beware of trying to soak up some heady material during exercise—like mastering a physics test while you're on the treadmill. Here's why: during exercise, the oxygen is shunted to other parts of the body where it is needed most. The brain benefits occur *after* you complete the workout and have your cool down. That might explain why you may find it impossible to concentrate on that very interesting book you brought with you to read while on the stationary bike at the gym. The time to hit the books is after the physical stress of exercise, not during.

Pillar 2: Proper Nutrition

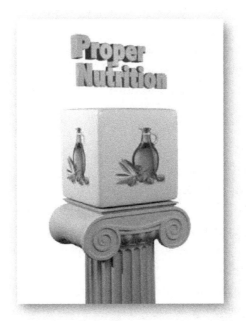

I N 1826, THE famous French gastronome Anthelme Brillat-Savarin wrote in his treatise, *Physiologie du Gout, ou Meditations de Gastronomie Transcendante*: "Tell me what you eat and I will tell you what you are."[18] And in 1863, in an essay titled *Concerning Spiritualism and Materialism*, Ludwig Andreas Feuerbach, a German philosopher, wrote, "man is what he eats."[19] Hence the

---

18 "Physiologie du Goût," Division of Rare and Manuscript Collections, Cornell University Library, 2002, http://rmc.library.cornell.edu/food/gastronomy/Physiologie_du_Gout_L.htm.
19 "The Meaning and Origin of the Expression: You Are What You Eat," Gary Martin, 2016, http://www.phrases.org.uk/meanings/you-are-what-you-eat.html.

phrase in common usage today, "You are what you eat"; and while the original phrase didn't mean it literally, there is much truth to that statement.

In our *Five Pillars of Brain Fitness* classes, we often ask participants: "How many of you think what you eat plays a role in the health of your brain?" Inevitably, all hands go up. But what exactly constitutes a brain-healthy diet?

How Nutrition Affects Brain Fitness

Your brain needs certain essential nutrients in order to function properly. These nutrients are classified as *macronutrients, micronutrients,* and *phytonutrients.* Macronutrients are needed in larger quantities and include water, proteins, carbohydrates, and lipids (fats). Micronutrients, needed in small quantities, consist of vitamins and minerals. Phytonutrients are trace chemicals found in plant matter.

Macronutrients

Your brain is mostly composed of two components: water and fat. Maintaining a proper water balance is vital for brain functioning. In February 2012, researchers at the University of Connecticut's Human Performance Laboratory discovered that mood and cognitive function could be adversely affected by even mild dehydration.

Too much water can be even more dangerous. Water intoxication, also known as *water poisoning* or *dilutional hyponatremia,*[20] is a potentially fatal disturbance in brain function that results when the normal balance of electrolytes in the body is pushed outside safe limits by over hydration. Water intoxication is a rare phenomenon usually brought on by a person either voluntarily or involuntarily consuming large quantities of liquid. Clearly, maintaining proper hydration levels is vital to maintaining your brain's health.

---

20 Jorge Garcia Leiva et al., "Pathophysiology of Ascites and Dilutional Hyponatremia: Contemporary Use of Aquaretic Agents," *Annals of Hepatology* 6, no. 4 (2007): 214–21.

Lipids

Lipids, commonly known as *fats*, comprise about two-thirds of your brain's tissue.[21] These lipids come in the form of fatty acids. The body cannot synthesize fatty acids, so we must get them from our diets. Fatty acids, also called *omega fatty acids*, are found in a variety of food substances, including tree nuts, flaxseeds, and some vegetables, such as soybeans, Brussels sprouts, and cauliflower. An excellent source of omega-3 fatty acids is fish, especially cold-water fatty fish, such as salmon, codfish, halibut, and sardines.

There are three primary types of fatty acids that are essential for human health:

- Alpha-linolenic acid (ALA)
- Eicosapentaenoic acid (EPA)
- Docosahexaenoic acid (DHA)

Of these, DHA is the superstar for brain health. In fact, your brain is mostly made up of DHA. As mentioned earlier, an excellent source of DHA is fish. If you're not a fan of fish, you can purchase a fish oil supplement at your local pharmacy, but be aware that not all fish oil supplements are the same.

The amount of DHA present in fish oil capsules varies widely from manufacturer to manufacturer. Ignore the milligram dosage on the front label and instead look at the ingredients label on the back of the bottle for the EPA and DHA concentrations. Also check to see how many capsules you need to take to get the listed amount of DHA. Figure 1 shows three different brands that differ widely in DHA content.

Brand A contains 120 mg in one softgel. Brand B contains 385 mg in one softgel—that's more than three times the amount contained in Brand A. Brand C lists DHA content as 600 mg, but you need to take three softgels to get the 600 mg, so each softgel actually contains 200 mg of DHA. Brand B contains the most per softgel, followed by brand C and then brand A.

---

21 Chia-Yu Chang, Der-Shin Ke, and Jen-Yin Chen, "Essential Fatty Acids and Human Brain," *Acta Neurologica Taiwanica* 18, no. 4 (2009): 231–41.

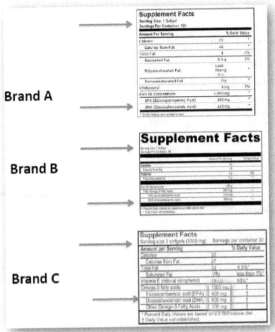

Figure 1. Comparison of DHA Content

For those who are vegans or vegetarians, there are DHA capsules made from algae oil instead of fish oil.

Carbohydrates

Carbohydrates are another important macronutrient for the brain. Carbohydrates provide more than 60 percent of the amount of energy required by the body. Carbohydrates come in two forms, simple and complex. Simple carbohydrates are basically types of sugar. There are many types of sugars that come from a variety of sources, such as sucrose (table sugar), which comes from sugar cane or sugar beets; fructose, which comes from plants; and lactose, which is found in milk. Sugars are simple forms of carbohydrates that are easily digested by most people. The exception is lactose, which some adults have difficulty digesting (lactose intolerance).

Complex carbohydrates are chemically more complex than simple carbohydrates, hence the name. Complex carbohydrates consist of a chemical structure that is made up of three or more sugars, which are usually linked together to form a chain. Complex carbohydrates can be rich in fiber, vitamins, and minerals. Due to their chemical complexity, they take a little longer to digest, and they don't raise blood sugar levels as quickly as simple carbohydrates. Complex carbohydrates act as the body's fuel, and they contribute significantly to energy production.

Simple Carbohydrates

There are two types of simple carbohydrates: monosaccharides and disaccharides. Monosaccharides consist of only one sugar; examples include fructose, galactose, and glucose. Disaccharides consist of two chemically linked monosaccharides. An example is sucrose (table sugar), which consists of one molecule of glucose and one molecule of fructose. The most important type of simple carbohydrate, or sugar, as far as the brain is concerned is glucose. Glucose is what the brain metabolizes to produce the energy it needs to function. The brain is the most energy-dependent organ in your body, consuming about 20 percent of all the energy your body requires. Without sufficient glucose in your bloodstream, brain cells start to atrophy and die.

As mentioned earlier, table sugar (sucrose) is a disaccharide consisting of one glucose molecule and one fructose molecule. When metabolized, the body breaks the bond between the two sugars. It uses the glucose molecule to produce energy (calories) and sends the fructose molecule to the liver, where it is further broken down and often stored in the liver and other tissue.

How Sugar Undermines Brain Health

Brain cells, and all the other cells in your body, rely on insulin to convert the glucose in your bloodstream into the energy required to power your brain cells. As we age, brain cells may begin to lose the ability to efficiently utilize insulin to metabolize sugar. They become insulin resistant. When this happens, brain cells begin to atrophy and die. This cellular insulin resistance in the brain is similar to what the body experiences in an individual with diabetes. In fact, some researchers are stating to refer to insulin resistance in the brain as *type 3 diabetes*.[22]

You likely know that chronic high insulin levels in the bloodstream can lead to diabetes, but did you know that diabetes more than doubles the risk of developing Alzheimer's disease? One study, published in the *Journal of Neurology*, followed one thousand adults for more than fifteen years. Over that time period, those diagnosed with diabetes had increased their risk of dementia by 74 percent.

Most Americans are in no danger of getting insufficient sugar in their daily diets. In fact, what do you suppose is the biggest source of calories in the American diet today? Fats? Sugars? Carbohydrates? If you answered sugar, you are correct. Sugar, especially in the form of high fructose corn syrup (HFCS), is ubiquitous in processed foods. It's clear that some products contain high levels of HFCS, but others are not so obvious. Did you know that apple juice, applesauce, ketchup, peanut butter, yogurt, salad dressings, processed cereals, energy bars, and many other products can contain high levels of HFCS? Shockingly, HFCS is even found in many infant formulas.[23]

A study published in the *Journal of the American Medical Association* found that most adults consumed 10 percent or more calories from added sugar, and approximately 10 percent consumed 25 percent or more.[24] Health risks were higher when comparing participants who consumed 25 percent or more calories from added sugar with those who consumed fewer than 10 percent of calories from added sugar. These findings were largely consistent across age group, sex, race/ethnicity, educational attainment, and physical activity. The researchers concluded that most US adults consume more added sugar than is recommended for a healthy diet. They observed

22 Suzanne M. de la Monte and Jack R. Wands, "Alzheimer's Disease Is Type 3 Diabetes—Evidence Reviewed," *Journal of Diabetes Science and Technology* 2, no. 6 (2008): 1101–13.
23 William Sears, "Corn Syrup in Formula," *Parenting*, 2016, http://www.parenting.com/article/corn-syrup-in-formula.
24 Quanhe Yang et al., "Added Sugar Intake and Cardiovascular Disease Mortality Among US Adults," *JAMA Internal Medicine* 174, no. 4 (2014): 516–24, doi:10.1001/jamainternmed.2013.13563.

a significant relationship between added sugar consumption and increased risk for cardiovascular disease mortality; thus, you can immediately improve your brain-healthy diet by limiting the amount of sugar, especially HFCS, in your diet.

See appendix 1 for more on sugar.

Complex Carbohydrates

Complex carbohydrates (starches) are typically found in fruits and vegetables. They are broken down into their constituent chemical components that include proteins, sugars, vitamins, minerals, phytonutrients, and indigestible fiber. Complex carbohydrates tend not to produce the same blood sugar spikes that sugars do, because the sugar contained in them enters the bloodstream more slowly. However, some complex-carbohydrate-rich foods can cause elevated blood sugar levels. Examples include potatoes, white rice, pastas, and bread made with processed flour. Overall, however, complex carbohydrates tend to be healthier than simple carbohydrates. The last section of this chapter on the Mediterranean diet discusses the nutritional content of complex-carbohydrate-rich foods in greater detail.

Proteins

Proteins contain amino acids, the building blocks for creating new cells, and are essential to every cellular function. Proteins are very large molecules made up of various amino acid chains. There are millions of types of proteins. Good sources of proteins for a brain-healthy diet include:

- Seafood
- White meat poultry
- Lean red meat in moderation
- Eggs
- Dairy products in moderation
- Soy
- Beans

Most Americans get adequate supplies of protein in their normal diets. However, a diet high in fatty red meats and dairy products, while providing healthful proteins, also can raise cholesterol and triglyceride levels, which can cause damage to brain cells.

Micronutrients

Vitamins and minerals in small quantities constitute the essential micronutrients. The brain requires a wide variety of vitamins and minerals to function properly; however, there are a few micronutrients that are especially important for maintaining a healthy brain.

The B vitamin group is crucial to brain fitness. Deficiencies in certain B vitamins can cause cognitive decline. Important B vitamins for brain function include thiamin (B1), niacin (B3), pantothenic acid (B5), pyridoxine (B6), biotin (B7), and cobalamin (B12). Vitamin B12 deficiency, which affects 10–15 percent of adults over the age of sixty, is frequently associated with neurological problems. As we age, our digestive tracts don't process B12 as efficiently as when we were young, so it is common to see B12 deficiencies in the elderly. Fortunately, taking B vitamin supplements can usually reverse cognitive loss due to B vitamin deficiency. In extreme cases, a B12 injection may be required.

Vitamin E is important for maintaining a healthy brain. Vitamin E is a powerful antioxidant that protects neurons from oxidative damage. Vitamin E deficiencies cause neurological symptoms, such as impaired balance and coordination, muscle weakness, and damage to the retina of the eye. Vitamin E is also crucial for proper neural development in infants.

Vitamin D is another essential brain micronutrient Vitamin D is important for normal brain development and function. Accordingly, vitamin D deficiency may impair cognitive abilities. Vitamin D deficiency is a major problem worldwide, with an estimated one billion people having insufficient or deficient levels of vitamin D. Aging is associated with a reduced capacity to synthesize vitamin D in the skin upon sun exposure. Thus, older adults may be more vulnerable to vitamin D deficiency and any untoward effects on cognition.

The brain relies on many other micronutrients to remain healthy. For most individuals, following a well-balanced, healthy diet provides all the micronutrients we need. But as we age, vitamin and mineral supplementation may be beneficial.

Phytonutrients

Phytonutrients, also called *phytochemicals*, are substances found in plants that help protect them from bacteria, fungi, and disease. Phytonutrients are considered a nonessential nutrient in the human diet; that is, they are not required in our diets for survival. However, researchers believe phytonutrients may play a beneficial role in fighting diseases in humans.

Many thousands of phytonutrients have been identified. Phytonutrients thought to have a beneficial effect for people fall into several general groups, such as:

- Carotenoids (a powerful class of antioxidants)
- Ellagic acid (protects against cancer)
- Flavonoids (help protect against cancer and heart disease)
- Resveratrol (antioxidant and anti-inflammatory)
- Glucosinolates (anticancer properties)
- Phytoestrogens (may have anticancer properties in women)

For a further discussion on phytonutrients, see appendix 3.

Which Diet Is Smarter: Mediterranean or Paleo?

Through consultations with dietitians, neurologists, and other brain researchers, we arrived at a clear consensus as to what constitutes a brain-healthy diet. Brain-healthy diets are:

- Low in saturated and trans fats (with one notable exception)
- High in mono- and polyunsaturated fats
- Low in simple carbohydrates and sugars
- High in fresh vegetables and fruits
- Include a moderate amount of whole grains, nuts, and seeds

- Include a moderate consumption of alcohol
- Include some vitamin and mineral supplements

Two diets that meet these criteria are the Mediterranean and Paleo diets. The Mediterranean diet features foods commonly consumed in countries surrounding the Mediterranean Sea. Dr. Walter Willett, Dr. Frank Sacks, and others originally created the Mediterranean diet at the Harvard School of Public Health.[25] Dr. Willett and Dr. Sacks suggest red meat either a few times a month or no more than one ounce a day, four to six ounces of poultry three or four times a week, and four to six ounces of fish three to seven times a week. The Mediterranean pyramid puts beans in a separate category with legumes and nuts and recommends that foods from this category be eaten daily. It also recommends daily physical activity and, optionally, that some wine be consumed daily.

The Paleo or Paleolithic diet is a nutritional plan based on the presumed diet of Paleolithic humans. It is based on the premise that human genetics have scarcely changed since the dawn of agriculture, which marked the end of the Paleolithic era ten thousand years ago. The Paleo diet consists mainly of fish; grass-fed, pasture-raised meats; eggs; vegetables; fruit; fungi; roots; and nuts. It excludes grains, legumes, dairy products, potatoes, refined salt, refined sugar, and processed oils.

At Brainstorm Mind Fitness, we recommend the Mediterranean diet because it's more flexible, easier to follow, and more palatable to most people's tastes than the Paleo diet. However, if you prefer the Paleo diet, by all means follow it. Each is a brain-smart way of eating.

Steps to a Healthier Plate

To summarize, avoid excess sugar, and get your carbs from raw or cooked vegetables, fruits, nuts, whole grains, and legumes. Also avoid processed carbohydrates, such as white bread, pasta, and white rice.

---

25 Marian Burrow, "Eating Well," *The New York Times,* March 29, 1995, http://www. nytimes.com/1989/11/15/garden/eating-well-marian-burros.html.

The next step is to limit red meats, such as beef, lamb, and pork, and replace them with poultry and seafood. Especially good are high-fat fish from cold waters, such as wild-caught salmon, codfish, halibut, mackerel, and sardines. Stay away from foods that are high in cholesterol or contain trans fats, hydrogenated oils, and saturated fats, such as processed and fast foods.

One exception to avoiding saturated fats is organic virgin coconut oil. Unprocessed virgin coconut oil seems to be processed differently by the body than other saturated fats. Coconut oil is a medium chain triglyceride that has received a lot of popular press coverage as having LDL-cholesterol-lowering and HDL-cholesterol-raising properties. It may also serve as an alternate fuel source for brain cells that have become resistant to insulin and can't metabolize blood sugar properly. While most of the evidence is anecdotal, we have seen some impressive results from adding a tablespoon a day of coconut oil to your diet.

Supplements

Most of us get adequate amounts of essential vitamins and minerals by following a healthy, well-balanced diet, such as the Mediterranean diet. However, as we age, we may need some vitamin and mineral supplementation. The US dietary supplements industry is huge, with annual sales in excess of $11 billion. The efficacy of dietary supplements varies from individual to individual, supplement to supplement, and manufacturer to manufacturer. Many dietary supplements are manufactured in China under questionable quality control standards. In one study, Canadian researchers tested forty-four herbal supplements and found that many contain ingredients that can cause problems for people with food allergies. In some cases, it was discovered that supplements did not contain the amounts of active ingredients that their labels claimed. Because the Food and Drug Administration does not regulate dietary supplements in the same way that prescription drugs are regulated, you are left to rely on the manufacturer's claims. This has led some to label the dietary supplement industry as "the Wild West of the drug-making industry." You can research supplement brands online, or ask for your health care provider's recommendation.

Because each individual is different, it is difficult to recommend across-the-board supplements. If necessary, your healthcare practitioner can order blood tests to determine if you have a micronutrient deficiency.

For more detail on nutritional supplements for cognition, see appendix 2.

Pillar 3: Mental Exercise

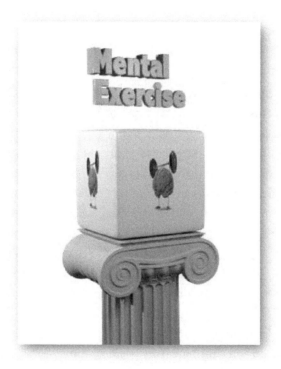

IN HIS EXCELLENT book *Keep Your Brain Alive*, Lawrence Katz coined the term "Neurobics" to describe mental exercises designed to keep one's brain agile and healthy. As he says in his book, "Neurobics aims to help you maintain a continuing level of mental fitness, strength, and flexibility as you age."

A neurobic exercise program that includes novel, non-routine mental exercises activates all of your senses to stimulate neural activity that in turn promotes the formation of new neural pathways. As new neural pathways are established, BDNF is produced in the brain. As described in previous sections, BDNF promotes synaptogenesis, which is the creation of new connections among neurons.

BDNF may also contribute to neurogenesis, or the growing of new brain cells. Contrary to what you may have heard, you are not born with a limited number of brain cells. We now know that it is possible for the brain to generate new neurons from neural stem cells in certain parts of the brain. One of those parts is the hippocampus, which plays a major role in short-term memory.

Memory

Most of us, at one time or another, have had the experience of forgetting a familiar name, misplacing your car keys, or walking into a room and being unable to remember why you went in there. Don't worry; forgetting is a normal part of being human. Imagine how cluttered your brain would be if you remembered absolutely everything you experienced. In fact, there are only a very few individuals who can remember in vivid detail every day of their

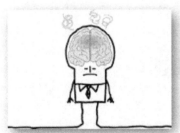

lives. Medical science has documented about twenty-six cases of *hyperthymesia*, the medical term used to describe this condition. Some individuals diagnosed with hyperthymesia report that the constant, irrepressible stream of memories has caused significant disruption to their lives.

At what age do you think memory peaks in most people? Studies vary, but in general it is thought that memory peaks on average somewhere between the ages of twenty-two and twenty-seven.[26] Keep in mind, that's when memory peaks, not intelligence and certainly not knowledge. In fact, the amount of

26 Joshua K. Hartshorn and Laura T. Germine, "When Does Cognitive Function Peak? The Asynchronous Rise and Fall of Different Cognitive Abilities Across the Life Span," *Psychological Science* 26, no. 4 (2015): 433–43, doi:10.1177/0956797614567339.

white matter in the brain, which forms the connections among nerve cells, seems to increase until age forty or fifty and then falls off again.

What causes forgetfulness? Memory slips are aggravating, frustrating, and sometimes worrisome. When they happen more than they should, they can trigger fears of looming dementia or Alzheimer's disease. However, many of the causes of forgetfulness are the result of normal processes. A Harvard Medical School journal cites seven common causes of forgetfulness. They include:

- Lack of sleep
- Certain medications
- Underactive thyroid (hypothyroidism)
- Alcohol
- Stress and anxiety
- Depression

We sometimes forget things because we're not paying attention. Have you ever attended a presentation and noticed people in the audience texting on their phones? You can bet they won't remember much of what's being said. Distractions can also cause forgetfulness, and we all have plenty of distractions on a daily basis in our modern lives.

How Memory Works

The way the brain forms and retrieves memories is a complex process involving many areas of the brain. To simplify things, you can think of memory formation as being a three-stage process.

First, information from the five senses enters the brain and is routed to the hippocampus, the area of the brain that processes short-term memory. Much, if not most, of this sensory information is discarded quickly because we're focused on something else. As the hippocampus sorts through the barrage of sensory information streaming in from moment to moment, the brain decides to hold on to some of this input for a short period of time. We call this *working memory*. Studies have shown that most people can only hold between five and nine pieces of information at a time in working memory, so the hippocampus has to make a decision on what to save to longer term memory and what to discard or forget. It has to do this quickly, too, because new information is pouring in constantly.

The hippocampus chooses certain bits of information it decides are important enough to save in a process called *encoding*. Once a piece of information has been encoded, a neural pathway to the prefrontal cortex is created. This is the second stage of memory called *consolidation,* or storage. At this point, the memory exists in both the hippocampus (short-term memory) and the prefrontal cortex (long-term memory).

A memory isn't really a memory until it is retrieved, and *retrieval* is the third stage of memory formation. It has been shown that the more times a memory is retrieved, the more resilient that memory becomes.

A strange thing has been discovered about these neural pathways of memory. Scientists conducting studies on mice and memory formations attached electrodes to a mouse's brain and then had the mouse learn a pathway in a maze. Using sophisticated brain imaging techniques, the researchers were able to "see" the neural pathway between the hippocampus and the prefrontal cortex of the mouse's brain. They could see the same neural pathway firing each time the mouse ran the maze.

Eventually, the mouse got tired and went to sleep. When the researchers looked at what was happening as the mouse slept, to their surprise, they saw that that same neural pathway that had just been formed while learning the maze was firing again and again as the mouse slept. Amazingly, the neural pathway fired thousands of times as the mouse slept. It seems that once we store a memory, we rehearse that memory in our sleep as a way of reinforcing the neural pathway of the memory.

Eventually, the neural pathway connection between the hippocampus and the prefrontal cortex is severed, and it is at this point that the memory is a "permanent" part of long-term memory. Studies have shown that it can take as long as ten years for this to occur.

The Scientific Basis of Neurobics

In the beginning of this chapter, we talked about the pivotal role of BDNF. This important molecule is secreted in the brain when our muscles exercise and when we create new neural pathways by learning something new. BDNF produced by physical exercise can promote neurogenesis (the growth of new brain cells), dendritic sprouting (growth), and synaptogenesis (connecting nodes between brain cells that transfer neural signals from one brain cell to the next) in some parts of the brain.

BDNF does not spur the development of new brain cells and connections in all parts of the brain. One area of the brain that is able to produce new neurons throughout life is the hippocampus, which contributes to memory formation.

Notice that when we refer to mental exercises that most benefit the brain, we refer to *novel* or *nonroutine* exercises. Learning something new produces new neural pathways and the secretion of more BDNF than simply repeating the same mental exercise day after day.

We frequently ask people attending our presentations if they keep their brains mentally active, and we often get responses such as "Oh, yes. I do the crossword puzzle every day," or "I do those Sudoku puzzles every day."

That's good, but you can do better. Doing those types of mental exercises each day is helpful but not as helpful as trying something completely new. Doing the same puzzles day after day may just mean that you are getting better at doing crossword puzzles but not necessarily at learning something new.

Another fun way to exercise neurobically is to utilize a sense in a novel way by *sense blunting*. For example, try blunting your sense of vision by wearing a blindfold and then try to identify various objects by touch or smell or taste. Do this exercise with a partner who can pick objects for you to identify while blindfolded. Make it more challenging by holding your nose while blindfolded and trying to identify different foods by taste alone. It's very difficult, because the sensation of taste relies heavily on your sense of smell. These exercises are especially fun to do with your children or grandchildren.

Three Neurobic Rules

Here are three rules to follow to get the most out of neurobic exercise:

1. Involve one or more of your senses in a novel, nonroutine context. Sense-blunting exercises work well for this

2. Engage your attention. To make your brain go into "alert" mode, an exercise should be fun, surprising, or have meaning for you.

3. Break a routine activity in an unexpected way. Take a new route to work or to church.

Today, there is a proliferation of websites that provide challenging and varied neurobic exercises for a monthly fee. There are many excellent books on mental activity and "puzzlers" to keep the mind sharp. But you don't necessarily need an Internet subscription, an app, or a book to create mentally stimulating exercises. You can make up your own for free. For starters, try the exercises that we've suggested at the end of this book.

We're often asked, "How often do I need to practice my mental exercises to see a benefit?" We offer the same advice as we do when asked the same question about physical exercise: as often as you can, but at least three times a week for thirty minutes or more. The key is to make brain exercise a habit. Schedule particular time slots in your weekly schedule for brain exercise, and find a partner if you can. It is more fun when two people exercise together.

For a month-long list of suggested mental activities, see appendix 4.

Pillar 4: Social Activity

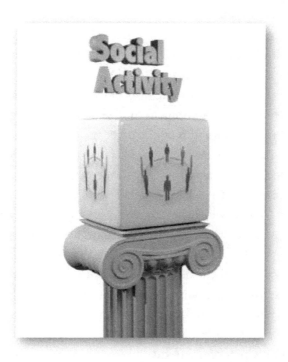

H UMANS ARE SOCIAL beings. Most healthy individuals prefer a socially active life rather than a solitary life. In fact, social isolation can be harmful to your body's mental and physical well-being. A 2013 study published in the *Proceedings of the National Academy of Sciences* suggests that being socially isolated may cause early death among the elderly. The research, which was led by Andrew Steptoe, a professor of epidemiology and public health at University College London, followed 6,500 British people over age fifty-two from 2004 until 2012.[27] The most socially isolated in this group were 26 percent more likely to die during the study period than those with the most active social lives, even after controlling for factors that also affect mortality, such as age and illness.

In a study of 2,249 California women published in the *American Journal of Public Health*, researchers reported that older women who maintained large social networks reduced their risk of dementia and delayed or prevented cognitive impairment.[28]

Individuals who were isolated as children display personality and learning disorders throughout much of their lives. At any stage of life, maintaining a socially active life helps to keep our brains and bodies healthy and fit.

Aging may cause many individuals to become more and more isolated for a variety of reasons. Diminished physical capabilities, such as impaired vision or hearing, difficulty with movement, problems with driving, fear of falling, or fear of embarrassment with cognitive decline, can be reasons for reduced social activity. In other cases, one member of a couple may develop health issues that place the other partner in a caregiver role, decreasing his or her ability to socialize. Often, social isolation is associated with increased states of depression and anxiety, which can become more common as we age. For all of these reasons and more, there is a tendency to become more isolated as we age.

Not only the elderly benefit from social interaction. Even otherwise healthy and active individuals can benefit from increased social activity. Social activities stimulate brain activity. Interacting with others on a regular basis promotes neurogenesis, dendritic branching, and healthy synaptic function. When you are socially active, you learn new things and experience new sensations, all of which promote the secretion of that brain-boosting protein BDNF, which nourishes brain cells.

27 Maia Szalavitz, "Social Isolation, Not Just Feeling Lonely, May Shorten Lives," *Time,* March 26, 2013, http://healthland.time.com/2013/03/26/social-isolation-not-just-feeling -lonely-may-shorten-lives/.

28 Michelle Diament, "How Friendship Keeps Our Brains Healthy," *Life Reimagined,* May 21, 2015, https://lifereimagined.aarp.org/stories/37251--How-Friendship-Keeps-Our-Brains-Healthy?cmp=SN-TWTTR-LR-POST-2015&sf38363302=1.

Researchers don't fully understand the correlation between socialization and brain health, but they have clearly established that there is a direct correlation between staying socially active and brain fitness. A 2011 study published in the journal *Nature Neuroscience* showed an increase in the volume of the amygdalae in the brains of study participants who maintained active social networks.[29] The amygdalae are small almond-shaped groups of nuclei in the medial temporal lobes of the brain that play a role in memory and emotions.

But staying socially active as we age can be a challenge, for reasons previously stated. Our best advice is to consider the barriers to keeping socially active and plan to overcome them. Find social situations and venues that are personally fulfilling. Set goals for social activities, such as participating in volunteer events, taking an adult education course, attending local performances, staying active in church, and the like. Transportation and personal mobility are big barriers to staying socially active; before driving skills become an issue, make sure you have researched public transportation options or connect with a friend or neighbor who may be able to give you an occasional lift. If personal mobility is an issue, investigate movement aids, such as canes, walkers, wheelchairs, and scooters. In many cases, Medicare will cover the cost of movement aids, as well as in-home physical and/or occupational therapy.

Humans are social animals. When you are engaged in a social activity, your brain is firing on all cylinders. It takes effort to remain socially active as we age, but the physical and mental benefits are well worth the effort, so get out your calendar and start planning some fun social activities for the weeks ahead.

29 Kevin C Bickart, Christopher I Wright, Rebecca J Dautoff, Bradford C Dickerson & Lisa Feldman Barrett Amygdala volume and social network size in humans Nature Neuroscience14,163–164(2011)doi:10.1038/nn.2724

Pillar 5: Stress Management

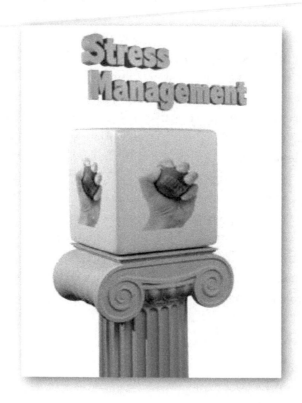

HAVE YOU EVER experienced the overwhelming sensation that your brain is free-falling into "shutdown" simply because you have too much going on at once? If you've ever muddled through a rough patch in your life, do you think of that time as a blur of events that are dimly remembered? Have you ever felt like your brain is so full of troubling details that you can't possibly learn anything new?

How about lying awake at night, tossing and turning, due to a worry that stubbornly occupies your thoughts? Or worse, losing sleep on a regular basis—so much that you depend on more and more cups of coffee just to get you going?

If so, you're not alone. In fact, you're with the majority. The World Health Organization now estimates that stress-related disorders affect nearly 450 million people worldwide. Some 80 percent of Americans report experiencing "intense, chronic stress" over personal finances and the economy.[30]

No matter how many self-help books are published every year, stress continues to plague the American population and lies at the root of troubling physical and psychological consequences. The most frequently cited sources of stress are work and money-related issues, but it can also result from commonly experienced life situations, including social and family issues, drug and alcohol abuse, isolation, and peer pressure.[31] Moreover, stress—or the perception of stress—varies from one person to another. What one person perceives as relaxing can be stressful to another; for example, a busy executive who enjoys his work may find vacation time frustrating and taxing.

Stress Damages: Body and Mind

Common physical symptoms that may be stress induced are elevated blood pressure, gastric ulcers, headaches, depression, and obesity. However, stress can also attack brain health, even potentially causing changes that impair cognition. As more scientists study memory and learning difficulties associated with forms of dementia, compelling evidence points to long-term stress as a major player in cerebral function or dysfunction.

In other words, if you've been under stress and your brain feels a little fuzzy, there may well be cause and effect playing out, unfortunately, in your head.

---

30 Richard J. Davidson, with Sharon Begley, *The Emotional Life of Your Brain: How Its Unique Patters Affect the Way You Think, Feel, and Live—and How You Can Change Them* (New York: Plume, 2013), 150–52.

31 "Stress in America: Paying with Our Health," American Psychological Association, February 4, 2015, http://www.apa.org/news/press/releases/stress/2014/stress-report.pdf.

The Wiring of the Stress Response

We react to stress in specific and purposeful ways, but the stress response generally has one ultimate intention: to save your life when threatened. The scientist Han Selye, an early and notable researcher, introduced the term *stress* and defined it as the "nonspecific response of the body to a demand." In the British Journal *Nature,* published in 1936, Selye called this reaction the *general adaptation syndrome,* or GAS, consisting of three stages: alarm reaction, resistance, and exhaustion.[32] The three stages are described as follows.

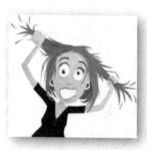

During the first stage of alarm reaction, the stressor activates the body, which prepares to fight or take flight. The body prepares for an emergency. Heart rate, respiration, and perspiration increase, and the pupils dilate. The stress hormones of adrenaline and cortisol are released. The body harnesses so much energy that the immune system is suppressed. You are ready for action!

In the resistance stage, the alarm reaction symptoms fade, allowing the immune system to bounce back. Hormones to reduce inflammation increase. Things return to normal. However, should the stressful stimuli or responses persist, the exhaustive stage follows—a point at which energy reserves are depleted. The body is not allowed to repair as it would in the resistance phase. Instead, the signs of the initial alarm reaction stay present without subsiding.

It's this final stage—the exhaustive stage—that poses the most trouble with brain health. And sadly, this type of stress, chronic and unrelenting, is the bane of our existence as we know it.

Stress as Part of Our World Today

Every year since 2011, the American Psychological Association has released a survey report called *Stress in America.* The study is comprehensive and inclusive of all ages—in fact, a troubling aspect of the latest report, published in 2014, was the revelation that teenagers now experience stress at reportedly higher

---

32 Carter, "Has Sleep and Stress Become a Vicious Cycle in Your Life?"

levels than adults. Both teens and adults report that their overall health suffers as a result of stress, manifested in unhealthy sleep, lack of exercise, and unwise eating habits. Here are some other depressing highlights from that study:

- Almost half (42 percent) of Americans say that their stress levels have increased in the past year.
- Even though the majority of Americans agree that stress management is important, few actually take the time to practice it.
- More than one-third (36 percent) of Americans report that stress affects their happiness "a great deal" or "a lot."

How Has the Stress Experience Changed?

From an evolutionary perspective, we still carry the same automatic stress response defenses that our cave-dwelling ancestors used for the fight-or-flight reaction. Just as a cat will arch its back or a deer will run away when encountering an unrecognized threat, this early response is intended for short-term use only.

In our world, however, most threats do not pose immediate physical harm. Instead, we experience the "smaller stressors" of work, deadlines, overdue bills, upcoming examinations, and the like. These brief stresses, however, can accumulate and become chronic, longer term catalysts for potential health problems. An overworked office employee, for example, may feel startled upon hearing the ring of the telephone or noticing the accumulation of unanswered e-mails.

In his excellent book, *Why Zebras Don't Get Ulcers*, Dr. Robert Sapolsky compares the way animals in the wild process stress to modern humans. Consider the reaction of the zebra when it sees a lion. The zebra's stress response to a predator is the same as a human's—the heart beats faster, the stress hormones kick into action, glucose is deployed into the blood, and oxygen is delivered to the extremities. But after things calm down and the zebra outruns the lion, it goes back to life as usual and homeostasis returns. For humans, however, the stress can be continual and unrelenting. Humans are still wired to cope with acute stress yet, unfortunately, lack the biological means to deal with sustained stress.

A Menu of Stress Types: Which One Are You?

Stress comes in different forms and intensities. The most common types are labeled *acute, episodic acute, chronic,* and *posttraumatic.*

Acute stress is the most common form of stress, stemming from perceived immediate demands and pressures. Do you enjoy rollerblading down a steep hill? Jumping out of small airplanes? Episodes of acute stress are thankfully short in duration and they don't come around often, so acute stress usually doesn't have time to create extensive damage.

Episodic acute stress affects individuals who suffer from acute stress on a recurring basis because of disordered, chaotic life circumstances. Although these individuals may be the unwitting victims of repeated stress in their environments—for example, civilians living in a war zone—many suffer because of self-inflicted behaviors. These are people who may describe themselves as type A personalities who take on too much and seem always in a hurry to try to meet their obligations. They may be easily aroused, short-tempered, irritable, and anxious. They react quickly with hostility if threatened or questioned.

Another episodic acute stress personality is a chronic worrier—that is, "worrywarts" who imagine that disaster is lurking around every corner and tend to predict catastrophe as an inevitable outcome. They tend to be tense and nervous and are commonly depressed.

Chronic stress is the everyday grinding stress that wears people out and is destructive to physical and mental health. It is created through the persistence of long-term problems, such as an unhappy marriage, despised job, or unrelenting poverty. In time, the sufferer of chronic stress will ignore the stress, tragically accepting it as "a way of life." Chronic stress symptoms are difficult to treat, even when the external aggravating circumstance is relieved.

Posttraumatic stress disorder is a distinct stress syndrome that we hear about frequently. It stems from traumatic experiences that become internalized and remain forever painful and present. Individuals experiencing posttraumatic stress disorder might exhibit signs of "hypervigilance" (like an easily triggered startle response). Loud noises, doors slamming, and shouting can set them off. They usually feel tense or on edge. In addition, PTSD sufferers frequently struggle with avoidance issues and feel they must stay away from places, events, or objects that are reminders of the experience.

Stress Triggers: A Myriad of Catalysts

The causes that pull the trigger for the stress response are many and varied. They can be external stresses, such as traffic jams, bad news, or an angry customer, or they can be internal stresses, such as the perception that work will never be caught up, a spouse will never change, or a child will always misbehave. Regardless of the source, the intensity of stress varies from person to person.

Emotional Stressors

Emotional stressors come in the form of fear and anxiety with general or global worries (Will there be more terrorist attacks?) or personal woes (What if I get laid off?"). They can present as a silent message given about our own shortcomings (I'm just awful at this, and I'm not going to do well.). People who expect the worst are "awfulizing" continually about tomorrow.

Social Stressors

Interaction with other people falls into the category of social stressor, and the degree of stress experienced in social situations can range from none to intense. Examples of common social stressors might include inviting someone out for a date, giving a public presentation, or having to approach a stranger in conversation. Some people might thrive in social situations, such as a party, while others would feel uncomfortable and dislike a crowded, unfamiliar situation.

Family Stressors

What was once the backbone of society—married couples with family and extended family that lived in close proximity to one another—has changed dramatically in recent decades. Nearly half of all marriages end in divorce, leaving more than 40 percent of all children spending part of their youth in single-parent households. Although the obvious stress of divorce is common, the very event of having children—even in solid marriages—presents complications and huge demands for adaptation for new parents. As children grow and change, so do the behaviors accompanying each development stage from toddlerhood to adolescence to early adulthood. In addition, many adults find themselves part of the sandwich generation, having to care for both their children and their aging parents.

Work Stressors

Stress at work is abundant. Like social stressors, it abounds in both paid and nonpaid workplaces and varies according to individual perception. While one person may find slow periods relaxing and deadlines stressful, another may be bored by routine work procedures, thriving only on higher levels of activity and deadline challenges. In recent years, with higher unemployment and limited opportunities in certain fields, many otherwise productive people are now subjected to the stress of unemployment or underemployment, finding themselves thwarted by an unhealthy economy.

Physical Stressors

Whenever we experience demands on our bodies so that physical health is compromised, we suffer the consequences. Examples of physical stresses include lack of adequate sleep, poor nutritional habits, or sustaining an injury from overusing a muscle in repetitive activity. Sufferers of chronic pain, gastrointestinal problems, or lack of alertness can expect to also incur mental stress from such conditions.

Disease Stressors

Disease stressors stem from both short-term and long-term disease, particularly the chronic diseases that people feel they have no control over, such as arthritis, allergies, diabetes, and asthma. Disease stress is not only experienced by the affected patient but also by the family members living with that person.

The Stress of Change and Decision-Making

Life changes, while they can be exciting and necessary, are also a powerful stress catalyst, erupting whenever anything of importance is altered in our lives. Examples of change stressors include moving to a new home, leaving a job, getting married, or traveling across the country to relocate to a new city.

The Feedback Loop of the Stress Response: How the Brain and the Body React

The stress response initiates a "feedback loop" governed by two systems with long (but mercifully abbreviated) names. Those systems are the *hypothalamic-pituitary-adrenal (HPA) axis* and the *sympathetic nervous system* (SNS). When activated by an area in the brain stem called the *locus coeruleus*, the SNS secretes the stress hormones called *epinephrine* and *norepinephrine*.

The HPA axis groups' stress responses are initiated by the pituitary and adrenal glands. Both the hypothalamus and the pituitary gland are involved with the slower maintenance response by signaling the adrenal cortex to release cortisol. As the stress hormones are released, the SNS kicks in to mobilize the body in response to perceived threats.

The path that stress takes throughout the body is large and generalized. If you've felt stressed to any degree, you may be aware that your body is responding with gusto—increasing your blood pressure and respirations. As your breathing becomes more labored, the digestive system slows down to shunt blood where it's needed, and the liver converts glycogen to glucose for fuel. Even the pupils dilate to give you more accurate vision, and your brain releases endogenous opiates to dull pain. You are like that zebra running from a lion!

More damaging, however, is the stress hormone cortisol that accompanies longer term, often emotional, stresses. Cortisol acts as a second line of defense and, although its effects are similar to adrenaline, such as elevating blood pressure, it actually undermines the very systems it was released to protect by gradual neuron receptor erosion. Thus, longer acting, emotionally based stressors can have devastating health consequences.[33]

---

33 Robert M. Sapolsky, *Why Zebras Don't Get Ulcers* (New York: Henry Holt, 2004), 16.

The Case of the Disappearing Hippocampus

As public and professional interest builds in the diseases affecting memory and thinking, such as Alzheimer's, research is being conducted on the consequences of stress in brain function and pathology. One of the primary structures involved in memory is the hippocampus.

The hippocampus is a small seahorse-shaped structure residing in the temporal lobe. Part of the limbic system, the hippocampus is positioned in both left- and right-brain hemispheres and is considered the gateway to new learning and consolidation of memory formation. Studies in the 1990s revealed that the hippocampus actually gathers memories from incoming sensory experiences and then assigns them to other parts of the cortex for long-term storage. In effect, the hippocampus's job is to turn short-term memories into long-term ones. One of the ways the hippocampus sorts through the sensory input it receives is through special receptors that interpret signals coming from outside the cells of the hippocampus. These receptors are how the hippocampus "hears" what's going on around it. Interestingly, it is one of the first brain structures to be damaged from Alzheimer's disease, which accounts for the common symptom of short-term memory loss.

The potential hazards of chronic stress on the hippocampus become more problematic over time; the longer the depression, stress, or trauma continues, the more the hippocampus shrinks and the more permanent the damage. Because the hippocampus has high levels of glucocorticoid receptors, it is particularly vulnerable to long-term stress. The stress hormones reduce excitability of neurons and suppress neuron regeneration. This damage, over time, creates atrophy and shrinkage of hippocampal volume. The longer the depression, the greater the shrinkage. It is not surprising, then, that adults who suffered from childhood trauma have a hippocampus that is 18 percent smaller than normal.[34]

---

34 Lise Gutkencht et al., "Tryptophan Hydroxylase-2 Gene Variation Influences Personality Traits and Disorders Related to Emotional Dysregulation," *The International Journal of Neuropsychopharmacology* 10, no. 3 (2007): 309–20.

The Brain on Stress: Depression, BDNF, and Learning

Recent studies have indicated that prolonged stress leads to the decrease of

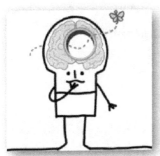

a healthy BDNF. As discussed elsewhere in this book, BDNF is a naturally occurring protein that helps to support neuron and synapse formation and is highly concentrated in the hippocampus. It has been associated with new learning and memory formation. However, the exposure to stress can actually suppress the expression of BDNF when overwhelmed by cortisol, as is the case with chronically depressed people. Thus, depression can make you a poor learner.

When Fear Won't Let Go: The Amygdala and Imprinted Memory

A key brain structure affected by stress, especially traumatic stress, is called the *amygdala*, an almond-shaped set of neurons residing in the middle temporal lobe close to the hippocampus. The amygdala is thought to be involved with modulation of memory formation associated with strong emotions.

Although the amygdala is connected with the prefrontal cortex, it is not a part of the conscious brain. It does not think through images or situations in a sophisticated way. Instead, it is part of the limbic system, an area that was well developed in animals before mankind arose, and is part of an active vigilance for survival.

This primitive part of the brain is thought to control the "fear response" by assessing the level of threat. Unfortunately, the amygdala can also be responsible for the memory of fear, even when out of danger. This theory has been supported by studies with rats. One study focused on new neurons formed in the hippocampus and the effect of a fear response created over a three-day period in a group of rats. The rats were confronted with the same fearful situation or a neutral yet novel situation the next day. When the researchers examined the rats' brains, they found that newborn neurons had been specifically activated by the fearful situation. However, when the amygdalae were destroyed, new neurons were no longer activated in response to the fearful memory.[35] This might explain why it is hard to shake a memory when it formed at the time of a highly charged emotional experience, as with veterans of war who "relive" an explosion years after the incident.

When Fear Trumps Rational Thinking

One of the correlations researchers have found among people with anxiety disorders is a smaller, more inactive prefrontal cortex—the part of the brain that should send the "stop signals" to the amygdala to halt the loop of anxiety symptoms. In effect, the prefrontal cortex isn't effectively interpreting the noise, so the amygdala takes over, tagging situations as survival threats and burning them as such into memory.

For example, you are driving home through a particular intersection when a car appears out of nowhere, running the stop sign and hitting you broadside, causing your car to swerve dangerously out of control. Even if you walk away unharmed by the accident, just passing the intersection in the future may cause you to feel nervous. In time, the fear becomes learned, and the circuit of a fear-related memory may become permanent.

Can Meditation Help? Resetting the Vagus Nerve

If you want to live life in a relatively calm state, you must have a healthy, fully functioning vagus nerve, a two-branch system running from the brain stem to the body across the abdomen and to the main organs, such as the heart and the stomach. Known in anatomy as the tenth cranial nerve, the vagus nerve controls the parasympathetic activity of the heart, lowering heart rate and respirations after a stressful event.

The opposing sympathetic system involves the opposite effect—gearing up the body for fight or flight. In tandem, the two systems work to offset each other, but when chronic stress is imposed, the parasympathetic system has little time to recover, if any. As a result, a person who lives with daily stress also

---

35 Kirby et al., "Basolateral Amygdala Regulation."

lives with higher levels of anxiety due to an underactive vagus nerve. When the vagus nerve is not fully functioning, the body loses its "reset button" to restore itself to a normal and alert sense of calmness.

Restoring the vagus nerve's calming effect may lie in the practice of meditation. In fact, an abundance of research supports the observation that practicing meditation and deep breathing may return the parasympathetic system and vagal tone to normal.[36]

In one study of meditation's effect on stress, university students were given a questionnaire to determine their anxiety levels in response to threats. Thirty-six of sixty-three students scored higher than normal; the remainder scored low. Then all the students were given a difficult math task with an imposed time limit to solve. After the test, they engaged in breathing and meditative exercise and returned to a state of calm. Heart rate and skin conductance were also measured to assess anxiety.

Those students who had higher levels of anxiety were more likely to have reduced vagal activity and lower heart rate variability after the stressful task, reflecting reduced responsiveness of the vagal nerve to the stressed environment. However, both groups (anxious and calmer) increased their heart rate variability after following the meditative and breathing exercises.[37]

Retraining Neural Pathways through Meditation

The success of meditation may have to do with "retraining" the neural pathways, overcoming the habitual ways of responding to challenges from past experience. Meditation or mindfulness training—involving attention to and focus on one's own thoughts—retrains the distress signals issued from the prefrontal cortex to calmer, more rational thoughts. Instead of heading to the amygdala part of the brain, which evokes a more fearful response, the neurons dissipate into other channels. As Dr. Richard Davidson so eloquently describes

---

36 Norman Doidge, *The Brain that Changes Itself: Stories of Personal Triumph from the Frontiers of Brain Science* (New York: Penguin Books, 2007), 241.

37 Narendra Singh et al., "An Overview on Ashwagandha: A Rasayana (Rejuvenator) of Ayurveda," *African Journal of Traditional, Complementary and Alternative Medicines* 8 (2011): 208–13, doi:10.4314/ajtcam.v8i5S.9.

in his book, *The Emotional Life of Your Brain,* "The more your thoughts travel along the path of less anxiety, the greater your reliance and the more positive your outlook."

Although meditative practices vary, most involve "deep breathing" or "belly breathing," which transports nitric oxide and dilates blood vessels and nasal passages. The pioneer of evoking a "relaxation response" as a response to stress is American cardiologist Dr. Herbert Benson. The steps to relaxation response are described in his seminal book, *The Relaxation Response.*[38]

1. Sit quietly in a comfortable position.
2. Close your eyes.
3. Deeply relax all your muscles, beginning at your feet and progressing up to your face. Keep them relaxed.
4. Breathe through your nose. Become aware of your breathing. As you breathe out, say the word "one" silently to yourself. For example, breathe in…out, "one," in…out, "one," and so on. Breathe easily and naturally.
5. Continue for ten to twenty minutes.

You may open your eyes to check the time, but do not use an alarm. When you finish, sit quietly for several minutes, at first with your eyes closed and later with your eyes open. Do not stand up for a few minutes.

Do not worry about whether you are successful in achieving a deep level of relaxation. Maintain a passive attitude and permit relaxation to occur at its own pace.

When distracting thoughts occur, try to ignore them by not dwelling on them, and return to repeating "one." With practice, the response should come with little effort. Practice the technique once or twice daily but not within two hours after any meal, as the digestive processes seem to interfere with the relaxation response.

---

38 Herbert Benson, *The Relaxation Response* (New York: Harper Torch, 1976), 162–63.

A Healthy Mind Needs Nightly ZZZZZs

We no longer think of sleeping as a pleasant snooze-fest activity but as a vital component of physical and mental health. The brain is actively engaged during the phases of sleep, and cognition can become impaired as people stay chronically sleep deprived.

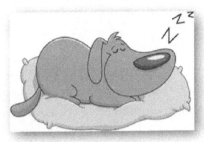

What goes awry when we don't get our nightly zzzzs? Too little sleep leaves us drowsy and unable to concentrate the next day. It also leads to impaired memory and physical performance and reduced ability to carry out math calculations. If sleep deprivation continues, hallucinations and mood swings may develop. Some experts believe that sleep gives the neurons we use while awake a chance to shut down and repair themselves. Sleep also may give the brain a chance to exercise important neuronal connections that might otherwise deteriorate from lack of activity.

Stress and sleep problems are strongly correlated. According to a survey by the National Sleep Foundation, more than two-thirds of women associate their sleep problems with stress. Yet more than half of the women polled said that sleep is the first thing they give up when running short of time. Without adequate sleep, the brain loses its opportunity to recharge itself through "sleep architecture," a relatively predictable pattern that occurs in ninety-minute cycles while we sleep. It involves an alternating pattern of rapid eye movement (REM) sleep and non-REM sleep.

REM sleep is an active sleep state where dreams occur, breathing and heart rate increase and become irregular, muscles relax, and eyes move back and forth under the eyelids. It's characterized by a high level of mental and physical activity where your heart rate, blood pressure, and breathing are very similar to what they are like when you're awake. Approximately 25 percent of total sleep time is spent in REM sleep, and it occurs about ninety minutes after falling asleep. REM sleep is vital, as it is the state that provides energy to the brain and body to help with performance throughout the day.

The other 75 percent of our sleep time is spent in non-REM sleep. Non-REM sleep has four distinct stages. Stage 1 is the beginning stage of feeling drowsy just as you're starting to doze off. In stage 2, the onset of actual sleep begins, and the body starts to adjust by lowering body temperature, while breathing and heart rate remain regular. Stages 3 and 4 are the deepest stages of sleep and provide our bodies with the best chance to restore what we used up during the daytime. During these stages, blood pressure drops, muscles relax, and breathing slows.

The number one rule of good sleep is keeping a routine: go to bed and get up at the same time, even on days off. A common temptation is to stay up late on days off, as the alarm clock isn't set for the next morning. But this is a sure way to throw off the sleep cycle, increasing tiredness when having to resume a different sleep/wake schedule on the first day back to work.

A relaxing bedtime routine, starting about an hour or more before you plan to go to bed, is another important part of sleep maintenance. Avoid stimulating activities: exercising, watching scary movies, reading mystery thrillers, or fretting with work issues on the computer. It takes time for the body and mind to settle down for sleep.

Other things to avoid in the evening hours before bedtime include heavy eating, caffeine, alcohol, and tobacco. Caffeine and tobacco keep you awake, and alcohol interferes with REM sleep.

The bedroom needs to be just that—a bedroom and not a place to work or watch television. At night, it's best to keep the room as dark as possible, as light inhibits sleep, so keep the shades drawn and forgo the night-light.

Nutrition and the Brain: Beyond the Pharmacy

Americans take record-breaking numbers of prescription medications to manage the problems attributed to stress. More than sixty million Americans take sleeping pills. One in ten take antidepressants.

Newer research points to nonprescriptive, natural alternatives to prescriptive medications that help individuals to overcome chronic problems with few side effects and risk of addiction. Such supplements include L-Theanine, lemon balm, 5-HTP, Ashwagandha, and melatonin.

L-Theanine: The Natural Calmer from Green Tea

Do you like to drink green tea? You may be surprised to learn that it has been known for centuries for its calming influence. That's because green tea contains L-Theanine, an amino acid that has specific effects on the brain and nervous system, helping to promote relaxation without the side effect of drowsiness.

Human studies have indicated that L-Theanine influences brain waves, inducing a calming and alert affect. In one study, subjects drank a soft drink containing green tea enriched with L-Theanine, while their brain wave power was measured. Initially, power was reduced in all frequencies, indicating relaxation. Later changes indicated increases in both relaxation and mental performance, suggesting that subjects could concentrate better with less anxiety.[39]

It should be noted that the amount of L-Theanine in a regular cup of caffeinated green tea is not large enough to produce adequate antianxiety effects, so supplementation is usually necessary. Most studies show benefits with doses between 100 and 250 mg per day. A cup of green tea contains less than 20 mg.

Lemon Balm

A common garden herb, lemon balm is known for its capacity to promote sleep; it is mildly sedate. Its primary components are rosmarinic acid, quercetrin, gallic acid, and rutin—powerful antioxidants that protect brain cells.

Lemon balm and rosmarinic acid are also boosters of the brain's relaxation-inducing neurotransmitter GABA, which inhibits the enzyme that reduces GABA. With increased amounts of GABA in the brain, anxiety is reduced.

Studies have been conducted using both animal and human subjects. In one study conducted at the Human Cognitive Neuroscience Unit at the University of Northumbria in the United Kingdom, researchers found that 600 mgs of lemon balm produced improvements in "accuracy of attention," while

---

39 David Eagleman, *Incognito: The Secret Lives of the Brain* (New York: Pantheon Books, 2011), 145.

300 mgs produced an increase in self-related reported calmness in a group of healthy adults. A later study using higher doses demonstrated significant improvements in both alertness and calmness using a singe 1600-mg dose.[40]

5-HTP

You may have heard of 5-HTP as an antidote for depression. That's because it is a precursor to serotonin, extracted from the Griffonia plant seed. 5-HTP (which stands for 5-Hydroxytryptophan) is an amino acid that easily crosses the blood–brain barrier and is then converted to serotonin.

Serotonin is the feel-good neurotransmitter primarily responsible for communication among cells; it is released and received throughout the brain and spinal cord. It is responsible for influencing numerous functions, including mood, movement, behavior, and eating patterns. When serotonin is low, symptoms of depression, anger, and aggression can arise, along with pain and addictive and compulsive behavior.[41]

The most common prescription drugs for depression fall into the category of drugs called *selective serotonin reuptake inhibitors*, or SSRIs. SSRIs prevent the presynaptic nerve from reabsorbing previously secreted serotonin. By inhibiting the absorption, an antidepressant of this category may cause an increase in serotonin without increasing the neurotransmitters.

Supplementing with 5-HTP increases the serotonin levels in the brain more naturally. Because it does not require a transporter, 5-HTP does not compete with other amino acids for absorption. The enzymes that breakc down tryptophan do not degrade it, and it is excreted through the kidneys.[42]

40 "Brain Basics: Understanding Sleep," National Institute of Neurological Disorders and Stroke, Last Modified July 25, 2014, http://www.ninds.nih.gov/disorders/brain_basics/understanding_sleep.htm.

41 Jay R. Kaplan et al., "Social Status, Environment and Atherosclerosis in Cynomolgus Monkeys," *Arteriosclerosis* 2, no. 5 (1982): 359–68, doi:10.1161/01.ATV.2.5.359.

42 Timothy C. Birdsall, "5-Hydroxytroptophan: A Clinically-Effective Serotonin Precursor," *Alternative Medicine Review* 3, no. 4 (1998): 271–80.

Ashwagandha

The herb Ashwagandha (*Withania somnifera*) grows in India, Pakistan, Afghanistan, Spain, Africa, the Middle East, and the Canary Islands. It is used as an adaptogen or tonic in Ayurvedic traditional medicine and is sometimes called *Indian ginseng*. The term *adaptogen* refers to an herbal substance designed to keep the body and mind "adaptable" to imposed circumstances. For years, Ashwagandha has been used in India as a tonic for many conditions, including stress relief, neuroprotection, analgesia, and inflammation. Today, Ashwagandha is being increasingly incorporated into natural formulas to restore the effects of stress.

Ashwagandha works as an anti-stressor by suppressing stress-induced increases of dopamine receptors in the brain. It also reduces stress-related increases of plasma corticosterone, blood urea nitrogen, and blood lactic acid. Like the antianxiety drug lorazepam, Ashwagandha was shown to reduce levels of tribulin, an endocoid marker of clinical anxiety, in rat brains when levels were increased by administering an axiogenic agent.

Adjusting the Body Clock with Melatonin

If you're subject to jet lag as a traveler, you may have tried melatonin, a substance naturally produced from tryptophan by the pineal gland. Melatonin is well known as a natural regulator of the body's daily biological rhythms. It works in conjunction with response to light and darkness through a special center of the hypothalamus called the *suprachiasmatic nucleus* (SCN).

The SCN works like a clock that sets off a regulated pattern of activities that affect the entire body. Once exposed to the first light of the day, the clock in the SCN begins performing functions, such as raising body temperature and releasing stimulating hormones like cortisol. The SCN also delays the release of other hormones, such as melatonin, which is associated with sleep onset, until hours later when the light fades. Production of melatonin is regulated by the body's pineal gland. This is a pea-sized gland located just above the middle of the brain. During the day, the pineal is inactive. When the sun goes down and darkness occurs, the pineal is "turned on" by the SCN and begins to actively produce melatonin, which is released into the bloodstream.

As a result, melatonin levels in the blood rise sharply, and you begin to feel less alert. Sleep becomes more inviting. Melatonin levels in the blood stay elevated for about twelve hours, until the light of a new day, when they fall back to low daytime levels by about 9:00 a.m. Daytime levels of melatonin are barely detectable.

Supplementation with melatonin has been shown to benefit the timing of sleep onset, sleep time, and quality. As a neuroprotectant, melatonin delivers antioxidants and helps to correct circadian rhythm, thus supporting cognitive function.

Cognitive Techniques: Can We "Out Think" Stress? Reframing

Can stress be managed in part by simply seeing the situation differently? This is the technique known as "reframing"—changing the way of looking at things by recognizing that there are many ways to interpret the situation at hand. The key is to rid negative thoughts and feelings that can result in stress. The shift might come from purposefully readjusting one's focus to the positive rather than the negative, spending less time in negative thought, and spending more time with people who are more upbeat in nature.

Positive Thinking: Is Stress a Choice?

Positive thinking has been a popular notion for decades. The idea is to rethink the usual destructive negative thought processes by focusing on strengths, learning from mistakes, and looking for opportunities. One suggestion in the realm of positive thinking is to realize that control of the situation is often up to the individual and changing the outcome is sometimes thwarted only by procrastination. In situations where there is truly no control over the outcome, the person is advised to let the situation resolve on its own without the needless worry and anxiety that usually accompanies the process.

Time Management

A common cause of stress can be the overwhelming feeling of being swamped and disorganized. A few tips to nip stress in the bud through better organization include:

- Keep a list of tasks in order of priority, and schedule a completion date for each.
- Start the day by identifying the most important task, and set about completing it first. That way, you're more likely to get things done.
- Learn to say no to projects not worth your time and energy. Saying, "I'd really like to do this, but I can't without giving up something else" is a good way to negotiate your time at work and at home.
- Allow yourself sufficient time to complete tasks. Realize that it usually takes longer than anticipated to complete tasks. A good rule of thumb is to always allow yourself 20 percent longer than you think necessary to meet a deadline.
- Segment your day accordingly. Hold off on answering calls, e-mails, and texts during the times you are focused, and stay on one task at a time.
- Plan the day to include breaks to physically or mentally take you away from the work at hand.
- Work stays at work; don't take it home unless absolutely necessary.
- If you work out of a home office, designate a particular space for working, and close it up at the end of the day.
- Control the timing of stressful events as much as you can. Trying to make decisions when you are rushed or anxious is difficult.

Venting to Others

People who keep things to themselves run the risk of stressing their brains without realizing it. In his book *Incognito*, Dr. David Eagleman cites a study at the University of Texas where long-held secrets went undiscussed with others, which included acting out of shame or guilt. The researchers concluded that when the subjects confessed or wrote about their secrets, their health improved, doctor visits decreased, and levels of stress hormones dropped.[43]

Seeking social support for problems, not necessarily to solve them but to air their burden, facilitates good health and morale. Support from family and friends or from professionals can help cushion the blow of a stressful event. An added suggestion is to journal about a frustration after talking about and then destroy it later so that rereading the journal will not reawaken the associated bad feeling.

Your Template for Stress Management: Where to Start

Understand how you stress. Everyone experiences stress differently. How do you know when you are stressed? How are your thoughts or behaviors different from times when you do not feel stressed?

Identify your sources of stress. What events or situations trigger stressful feelings? Are they related to your children, family, health, financial decisions, work, relationships, or something else?

Learn your own stress signals. People experience stress in different ways. You may have a hard time concentrating or making decisions; feel angry, irritable, or out of control; or experience headaches, muscle tension, or a lack of energy. Gauge your stress signals.

Recognize how you deal with stress. Determine if you are using unhealthy behaviors (such as smoking, drinking alcohol, and over/undereating) to cope. Is this a routine behavior, or is it specific to certain events or situations? Do you make unhealthy choices as a result of feeling rushed and overwhelmed?

Find healthy ways to manage stress. Consider healthy, stress-reducing activities, such as meditation, exercising, or talking things out with friends or family. Keep in mind that unhealthy behaviors develop over time and can be difficult to change. Don't take on too much at once. Focus on changing only one behavior at a time.

---

43 Ananya Mandal, "Hippocampus Functions," *News Medical,* January 14, 2014. http://www.news-medical.net/health/Hippocampus-Functions.aspx.

Take care of yourself. Eat right, get enough sleep, drink plenty of water, and engage in regular physical activity. Ensure that you have a healthy mind and body through activities such as yoga, taking walks, going to the gym, or playing sports that will enhance both your physical and mental health. Take regular vacations or other breaks from work. No matter how hectic life gets, make time for yourself—even if it's just for simple things like reading a good book or listening to your favorite music.

Reach out for support. Accepting help from supportive friends and family can improve your ability to manage stress. If you continue to feel overwhelmed by stress, you may want to talk to a psychologist, who can help you better manage stress and change unhealthy behavior.

Putting It all Together

OK, so now that you know all about the *Five Pillars of Brain Fitness*, what's next?

Well, that depends on why you read this book and what you learned about your own brain fitness. Readers tend to fall into three categories:

1. It looks like I'm doing most of the things suggested. I picked up a few new concepts, which I'll incorporate into my current lifestyle, but overall, I'm in pretty good shape.
2. I'm OK in some areas but way off on others. I'd better plan on changing my current habits.
3. Hmm. No wonder I can't remember to turn off the stove or where I parked my car.

Some readers will fit into category 1. Congratulations. You're already on the path to optimal brain fitness. Keep up the good work and maybe consider passing this book on to someone who might benefit from following the *Five Pillars of Brain Fitness.*

Many young people are interested in healthy lifestyles and likely fit into category 2. Maybe you work out regularly and eat a well-balanced diet, but you have a high level of stress in your life and have fallen into a bit of a neurobic rut. Having read the book, you likely have a good idea of the lifestyle strategies on which you need to focus.

If you fall into category 3, take heart. Progress is made in baby steps. Take the first step by starting somewhere, and then add more changes to your lifestyle. This is a marathon, not a sprint. The following pages contain ideas on setting goals and writing your own brain-health program.

Setting Goals

Start your goal setting with your highest priority, which may be your biggest weakness. Which pillar do you need to address the most?

Let's say, for example, that you are guilty of being mostly sedentary and that the only physical exercise you get is walking from the living room to the kitchen and occasionally lifting the remote control to the television. Your goal is to get more exercise, but how, exactly?

To answer this question, keep in mind that your goal must be *reasonable* and *specific.* Reasonable means that the goal is achievable and realistic, such as walking for fifteen minutes rather than running fifteen miles. Making that effort specific is to determine when, where, and how often you're going to walk. An example might be deciding to walk for fifteen minutes during your lunch break in the neighborhood behind your office five days a week.

Now go to your second highest priority and create a reasonable, specific goal for it. Again, focus on what you're missing and don't feel that you have to reinvent yourself overnight. As you progress and meet goals, it gets easier to enhance your program. The key is sticking to it and measuring your progress by creating a system of accountability. Read on.

Measuring Progress

A simple way to measure progress is to keep a daily chart of your brain-health endeavors and cross them off when completed. A sample progress chart is provided in appendix 7 to help you get started. Again, address the highest needs first, and tailor your chart accordingly. If your diet is really good but you are cheating yourself on sleep and have little interaction with others outside of work, then you need to work on rest and socialization. As you become more "accomplished" in certain areas—and the activity becomes too "easy"—challenge yourself by revising the goal. Bump up the exercise a notch, or tackle a different kind of brain game.

Rebooting

Things happen, and we all stray from the path from time to time. If you digress, you may need to reboot yourself and try again. We suggest examining what deters you from following through on your brain-health plan. Is it inconvenient? Is there no one to motivate you? Is the weather keeping you from your daily walk? Do you simply forget and fall back into old habits? When you look at the deterrents, you may have to revise your plan to something more realistic or add some sort of motivation element (e.g., an exercise partner) to keep you on track.

When you find yourself making excuses for not making time for brain-health practices, ask yourself this: What could possibly be more important than taking your full cognition with you for the rest of your years? Don't you deserve the effort and time it may take to maintain, regain, or improve the most important part of your being—your brain?

Appendix 1: The Sugar Wars

PARTICIPANTS AT OUR presentations will often say, "I understand that I should limit my intake of sugar, but when I do use sugar, which type is the healthiest: table sugar, turbinado sugar, honey, or agave syrup?"

Turbinado sugar, honey, and agave syrup are popular with the health-food crowd, especially agave syrup because of its low glycemic index, making it less likely to promote spikes in blood sugar.

We've read dozens of articles, some scholarly and some in the lay press, about sugar metabolism and the health effects of various types of sugar to determine if turbinado sugar, agave syrup, or honey is a healthier sweetener than sucrose (table sugar) or the dreaded high fructose corn syrup (HFCS), which is omnipresent in so many of our processed foods (it's even in baby formula).[44]

The first thing to know is that sugars come in several different molecular forms. Monosaccharides (single-molecule sugars) include glucose, fructose, and galactose. Polysaccharides (two-molecule sugars) include sucrose (fructose and glucose), lactose (glucose and galactose), and maltose (two glucose molecules).

After much research and consideration, it seems to come down to this: sugar is an important macronutrient, but too much sugar is a very, very bad thing regardless of the type. The main point is that we get too much of it in our processed-food diets.

It appears that the best type of sugar nutritionally is glucose (called *dextrose* commercially), because it is readily metabolized and quickly available for energy, or it is converted to glycogen that is then stored in the liver and muscle tissue. However, because glucose is readily metabolized in healthy bodies, too

---

44 Sears, "Corn Syrup in Formula."

much too fast can cause spikes in blood sugar that can lead to insulin resistance and diabetes.

Fructose appears to be the worst from a nutritional standpoint. We point out in our presentations that fructose largely bypasses insulin metabolism and goes straight to the liver, where it boosts blood triglyceride levels (hypertriglyceridemia) and is then converted into fat, which tends to get deposited in the abdomen. This can lead to increased risk of cardiovascular and kidney diseases and other maladies, such as obesity and diabetes. However, because fructose bypasses insulin metabolism, it has a low glycemic index and doesn't cause blood sugar spikes like glucose. For this reason, some people say it's a healthier sugar, but this ignores its hypertriglyceridemia and fat-producing aspects.

Pure agave syrup is about 90 percent fructose and 10 percent glucose, but processed agave syrups may include additional glucose, so the ratio is actually around 55–65 percent fructose. Honey contains fructose and glucose in about the same ratio. HFCS is about 55 percent fructose and 45 percent glucose. Sucrose (table sugar) is 50 percent glucose and 50 percent fructose. Turbinado sugar is basically sucrose that is less processed than white table sugar. Agave syrup and honey have the advantage of being less processed than HFCS, which is mostly produced from genetically modified corn and subjected to many pesticides and herbicides. Turbinado, honey, and agave also contain some vitamins, phytonutrients, and flavonoids not found in pure processed sugars.

In summary, glucose is easily metabolized and doesn't have the harmful effects that fructose does, but it may produce harmful blood sugar spikes. Fructose has a low glycemic index and doesn't produce blood sugar spikes, but it has the harmful effect of largely going straight to the liver, causing hypertriglyceridemia and producing unhealthy fats. With either sugar, there are advantages and disadvantages.

Conclusion: whether it's fructose or glucose, HFCS, agave, honey, turbinado, or table sugar, sugar in large quantities is harmful. The best advice is to limit the amount of added sugar in our diets, especially from processed foods containing HFCS. Ideally, we should try to get all the sugar we need (and we do need some in our diet) from fresh fruits and vegetables. In our humble opinion, it's a tie in the sugar wars.

Appendix 2: Nutritional Supplements and Cognition

DHA

DHA (DOCOSAHEXAENOIC ACID) is one of the essential omega-3 fatty acids commonly found in fish oil supplements. As you've read in this book, eating certain types of cold-water fish, such as salmon, tuna, mackerel, halibut, and herring, promotes a healthy brain, as they are primary sources of DHA.

DHA is "conditionally essential," which means that most of it must be obtained from food or dietary supplements, because it can't be synthesized in the body. That's because the body's method of synthesis is inefficient, and it takes a long time to produce enough to satisfy cellular needs. The good news is that if you take DHA by food or by supplement, it can be readily incorporated into cells.

DHA is the most abundant structural fatty acid in the brain and nervous system, playing a vital role in both prenatal and postnatal brain development. In fact, some research suggests that infants who receive DHA supplemented through breast milk score significantly better on mental and psychomotor development tests and that DHA may support normal activity levels and learning throughout preschool.

In adults, DHA plays many roles related to healthy cognition and memory. Studies over many years have documented that older adults have improved learning, memory, and problem solving when supplemented with DHA. One Dutch study monitored the dietary habits of a large group of elderly men over a period of three years. The researchers concluded that a high intake of cold-water fish was inversely correlated with cognitive impairment.[45]

Additional research has shown that low serum DHA levels are a significant risk factor for the development of Alzheimer's disease. Consistent observation reveals that the brains of Alzheimer's disease patients typically have a lower DHA content than the brains of normal adults of the same age.[46]

Along with protecting the brain from dementia, DHA seems to help with symptoms of depression. Research has demonstrated that depression is more common in patients with omega-3 fatty acid deficiencies and, not surprisingly, countries with the lowest consumption of fish tend to have the highest rates of depression. When depressed individuals were instructed to increase their fish intake over a period of five years, the incidence of depression decreased dramatically.[47]

Vitamin B12

Vitamin B12 is necessary for maintaining the integrity and function of nerve cells, promoting new cell synthesis, and supporting healthy nerve cell function. Although it is essential, it is the most common vitamin deficiency in the United States, particularly among seniors.[48]

The reasons for deficiency are wide and varied, but some common causes include the following:

- Poor absorption of oral vitamin B12, because the acidic content of the esophagus decreases with age.

---

45 S. Kalmijn, et al., "Polyunsaturated Fatty Acids, Antioxidants, and Cognitive Function in Very Old Men," *American Journal of Epidemiology* 145, no. 1 (1996): 33–41, doi:10.1093/oxfordjournals.aje.a009029.

46 Julie A. Conquer et al.. "Fatty Acid Analysis of Blood Plasma of Patients with Alzheimer's Disease, Other Types of Dementia, and Cognitive Impairment," *Lipids* 35, no. 12 (2000): 1305–12.

47 Lloyd A. Horrocks and Young K. Yeo, "Health Benefits of Docosahexaenoic Acid (DHA)," *Pharmacological Research* 40, no. 3 (1999): 211–25, doi:10.1006/phrs.1999.0495.

48 T. S. Dharmarajan, G. U. Adiga, and Edward P. Norkus, "Vitamin B12 Deficiency. Recognizing Subtle Symptoms in Older Adults," *Geriatrics* 58, no. 3 (2003): 37–8.

- A vegan or vegetarian diet, because B12 is derived from animal sources (including dairy and eggs).
- Interaction with commonly used medications, including metformin and common acid-suppressing drugs, that suppress absorption.
- Rarely screened as a routine test by physicians.

Symptoms of low B12 levels are plentiful and may include fatigue, lethargy, mood disturbances, and sluggishness. But major deficiencies can mimic more serious disorders, including dementia, depression, anxiety, and learning disorders.

The work of vitamin B12 is vital at the cellular level. Along with folate, vitamin B12 is involved in the synthesis of DNA and red blood cells. It also helps produce the insulation surrounding nerve cells, known as the *myelin sheath*. Think of the myelin sheath as the wrapper protecting the wires connecting the brain and nervous system.

If you suspect you have a B12 deficiency, get a blood test from your practitioner or from an independent lab. If you are B12 deficient, you may need help from a medical professional to determine the reason for the deficiency and to recommend the appropriate form and dose of supplementation.

Turmeric

The yellow-pigmented curry spice often used in Indian cuisine is a surprising source of brain and general health booster properties. Turmeric contains the bioactive ingredient curcumin, which is capable of crossing the blood–brain barrier—one reason why it seems to play a role in neurological disorders like Alzheimer's. Incidence of Alzheimer's in India is markedly lower than in the United States, a country where turmeric is eaten regularly with curry. It has been suggested that regular consumption of curry can lower or prevent Alzheimer's.

Research has suggested that curcumin may help inhibit the accumulation of destructive beta-amyloids in the brains of Alzheimer's patients, as well as aid in breaking up existing beta-amyloid plaques. Researchers from UCLA, the University of California, Riverside, and the Human BioMolecular Research

Institute have found that vitamin D3 plus curcumin may help stimulate the immune system to clear the brain of beta amyloids, which form the plaques. That study was published in the July 2009 issue of the *Journal of Alzheimer's Disease.*

Curcumin is also a powerful anti-inflammatory agent. Because people with Alzheimer's have higher levels of inflammation in their brains, it may play a role in inhibiting such inflammation.

Vitamin D

Although vitamin D is abundant in sunshine and in supplemental form, age-related decline in vitamin D, referred to as *hypovitaminosis D* (HVD), is common. Studies indicate that at least 40 percent, perhaps as high as 90 percent, of older adults have HVD, even those who live in sunny areas such as Florida.[49]

Because vitamin D is fat soluble, many elderly people (who often have a higher fat-to-muscle ratio) may retain more of the nutrient in fatty tissue and have less of it available in the blood to maintain proper health. In addition, as we age, our skin becomes less efficient at making vitamin D from the sun.

A review of the research on vitamin D deficiency and mental disorders at the University of Miami found five studies reporting an association between HVD and dementia, four studies linking it to mood disorders such as depression and bipolar disorder, and four studies linking it to schizophrenia.[50]

The bulk of the evidence so far suggests that people who have HVD are at greater risk for conditions such as stroke, dementia, and mood disorders than those who do not. What is not clear is whether short-term oral vitamin D supplements would reverse these conditions in people who already have them.

Defining the optimal dosage of oral vitamin D is tricky. A vitamin D-level blood test can indicate whether a person is at risk for deficiency and can be treated with supplementation under the guidance of a medical professional.

---

49 E. Paul Cherniack et al., "Hypovitaminosis D in the Elderly: From Bone to Brain," *The Journal of Nutrition Health and Aging* 12, no. 6 (2008): 366–73.

50 E. Paul Cherniack et al., "Some New Food for Thought: The Role of Vitamin D in the Mental Health of Older Adults," *Current Psychiatry Reports* 11, no. 12 (2009): 12–19.

In general, scientific evidence from animal studies shows that vitamin D supports healthy brain function throughout life. Vitamin D appears to be a "multipotent" brain cell-protective hormone, working through diverse and complex mechanisms, including brain calcium regulation, anti-oxidative properties, immune system regulation, and enhanced brain cell signaling.[51]

Vinpocetine

Vinpocetine is an extract from the seeds of the periwinkle plant (*Vinca minor*), a common, vine-like evergreen ground cover. It has a long history of use as a traditional tonic to alleviate weariness, especially the type associated with advanced age, and also as an astringent for excessive menses, bleeding gums, mouth sores, and more.

There are many ingredients in *Vinca minor,* but vinpocetine is the most interesting. Hundreds of studies of vinpocetine have been conducted with lab animals and human subjects. Vinpocetine is a derivative of the alkaloid vincamine, a substance that has been used to treat senile dementia. Studies of vinpocetine demonstrate many of the same functions as those of vincamine but without side effects. Moreover, it has been shown to be at least two times more potent than vincamine for improving cerebral circulation, memory, and other functions in humans. No interactions with pharmaceutical drugs have been reported.

In supplement form, vinpocetine helps memory by facilitating cerebral metabolism and improving blood flow in the brain. It works by causing mild dilation of blood vessels, thereby allowing for increased cerebral blood flow, which results in increased oxygenation and glucose utilization. In addition to enhancing brain circulation, vinpocetine has been found to increase brain-cell energy through its effect on the production of ATP (the cellular energy molecule).

Most studies showing positive benefits from vinpocetine have been done at amounts of 10 to 30 mg/day and some at 40 mg/day. All studies done at 30 mg/day showed additional benefits compared with lesser daily amounts, so

---

51 Stephen J. Kiraly et al., "Vitamin D as a Neuroactive Substance: Review," *Scientific World Journal* 26, no. 6 (2006): 125–39, doi:10.1100/tsw.2006.25.

this might be considered a starter dose. Please note that many cognitive formulas include vinpocetine as an ingredient, so be sure to check the individual dosage contained by reading the formula label carefully.

Huperzine

Huperzine A, a compound derived from the Huperzia serrata plant, is promoted as a memory enhancer because it acts as a cholinesterase inhibitor, meaning that it has similar effects on neurotransmitters as some FDA-approved drugs used for Alzheimer's disease. These effects include an increase in levels of acetylcholine, one of the chemicals that nerves use to communicate in the brain and elsewhere in the body. However, the first large-scale US clinical trial of huperzine A as a treatment for moderate Alzheimer's disease found that it provided no greater benefit than a placebo. Smaller studies have shown some improvements in memory and thinking in Alzheimer's patients with short-term treatment (duration of eight weeks).

In terms of memory enhancement, an older, small study published in the Chinese journal *Acta Pharmacologica Sinica* in 1999 found that huperzine A helped improve memory and learning in a group of adolescent students. For this study, sixty-eight junior high students (all of whom complained of memory inadequacy) were given either huperzine A or a placebo every day for four weeks. By the study's end, members of the huperzine A group showed greater improvements in learning and memory compared to members of the placebo group. Clearly, more and larger studies are needed to confirm huperzine's effectiveness as a safe memory aid. Studies are under way to test huperzine's effectiveness as a supplement for memory problems, including trials to investigate the effects of combining huperzine A with other drugs for Alzheimer's treatment. The hope is that these combinations may prove more effective than the pharmaceutical treatments that are currently available.

Coconut Oil

We are regularly asked about using coconut oil as a dietary supplement to support brain function, and the Internet is replete with stories of astonishing recoveries from memory disorders upon incorporating coconut oil into the daily diet.

The coconut oil benefit seems to come from ketones, the substance your body produces when it converts *fat* (as opposed to glucose) into energy. Primary sources of ketone bodies are the medium-chain triglycerides (MCT) found in coconut oil. Coconut oil contains about 66 percent MCTs. Your body does not process MCTs in the same manner as long-chain triglycerides. Normally, a fat taken into your body must be mixed with bile released from your gallbladder before it can be broken down in your digestive system.

But MCTs go directly to your liver, which naturally converts the oil into ketones, bypassing the bile entirely. Your liver then immediately releases the ketones into your bloodstream, where they are transported to your brain to be readily used as fuel.

Unlike glucose, some evidence suggests that ketone bodies may actually help restore and renew neurons and nerve function in the brain, even after damage has set in. Better yet, although the body treats MCT ketones as a carbohydrate rather than as a fat, there is no insulin spike from coconut oil.

Although more research is needed on coconut oil, a generally accepted "therapeutic dose" is 1–2 tablespoons (or 20 grams) a day. Because people tolerate coconut oil differently, it's a good idea to start slowly. Try one tablespoon and build up gradually. It's best to take it with food to avoid stomach upset.

Appendix 3: Phytonutrients

Besides the basic components of nutrition (vegetables, grains, legumes, herbs, nuts), there are beneficial substances in plants called *phytonutrients*. Scientists have identified tens of thousands of phytonutrients (also called *phytochemicals*). These chemical compounds help protect plants from injury and disease. Certain classes of phytonutrients have beneficial properties for humans, such as antioxidants and stroke and cancer-fighting properties. We'll look briefly at six classes of phytonutrients with healthful benefits. They are carotenoids, ellagic acid, flavonoids, glucosinolates, phytoestrogens, and resveratrol.

Carotenoids produce the orange, red, and yellow colors in fruits and vegetables. Carotenoids have antioxidant properties that help rid your body of harmful inflammation-causing free radicals. The carotenoid beta-carotene is converted to vitamin A in your body, which promotes good eye health. Carrots are a common source of beta-carotene. Lycopene, which imparts a red color in tomatoes and watermelon, is thought to help protect the body from prostate cancer. Lutein may help prevent eye problems, such as macular degeneration and cataracts, and is found in greens such as kale, collard, and spinach.

Ellagic acid is found in certain berries, such as strawberries, raspberries, and pomegranates. Ellagic acid is thought to have cancer-fighting properties.

Flavonoids are a large class of phytonutrients. They include catechins, which are found in green tea and thought to have cancer-fighting properties, and flavonols, which are found in apples and berries and might help fight coronary artery disease and asthma.

Glucosinolates, found in the cruciferous vegetables such as cabbage, broccoli, and kale, are thought to have cancer-fighting properties.

Phytoestrogens from soy foods may lower the risk of endometrial cancer and bone loss.

And lastly, one of our favorite phytonutrients is resveratrol, an antioxidant and anti-inflammatory compound found in grapes, grape juice, and, best of all, red wine. Resveratrol is thought to have cardiovascular and cancer-fighting properties and may even help extend life.

There are many other classes of phytonutrients, and researchers continue to discover more as interest in the health-promoting properties of phytonutrients grows.

Although phytonutrients are classified as nonessential nutrients, it just may turn out that they contain the key to a long and healthy life, so follow your mom's good advice and eat your fruits and vegetables.

Appendix 4: Daily Brain Exercises

Day 1: Speed up your brain's processing with sorting exercises.

THOROUGHLY SHUFFLE A deck of cards. Start a timer or a stopwatch. Sort the cards into the four suits: hearts, diamonds, spades, and clubs. (The cards don't have to be in order; just make four piles as quickly as you can.) How much time did that take you? Now try it again and see if you can beat that time. Hint: the key is to focus and try to block out extraneous thoughts while completing a manual, repetitive task. If you do not have a deck of cards on hand, you can substitute something else to sort, such as different types of dried beans, colored marbles, or jellybeans.

Day 2: Cue your memory with paired associative learning.

This exercise involves linking groups of words together and then memorizing them in pairs. It is an excellent exercise for rehearsing declarative memory, or how we provide the context in which we place memory content.

Memorize the following pairs of words in a few minutes. Try to link the words together so that when you hear "moon" you say "frog" (perhaps by visualizing a frog jumping over the moon).

Moon/Frog
Candle/Watchtower
Flower/Leaf
Road/Luggage

Radio/Computer

Now, **without looking**, write in the word associated with each word pair in the following space:

Moon/_____

Candle/_____

Flower/_____

Road/_____

Radio/_____

Day 3: Blunt a sense and heighten another.

One of the tenets of neurobics is to involve the senses to stimulate cognition. Today's exercise involves taking away the sense of sight while tasting food items. You'll need a partner and a blindfold as well as several types of chopped fruits. We like to use small pieces of melon, strawberries, kiwis, and raisins. While blindfolded, see if you can correctly identify the food that your partner feeds you on a toothpick. It's harder than it sounds!

Day 4: Master the name game.

Are you frequently searching for the name of someone you should know, be it a personal acquaintance or a movie star? Much of the trick with remembering names is to create visual or verbal strategies while learning them. For example, if you meet someone named Margie Monroe, try visualizing melting **margarine** on Marilyn **Monroe.** The sillier or more absurd the image, the more likely you are to remember the full name. Here's a list of names to practice with:

Jerry Finder

Mark Hill

Sandy Fairbanks

Dorothy Landsman

Chelsea Smart

Use a phonebook to make it more challenging, and select names randomly to see how fast you can create an association.

Day 5: Go backward and forward.

Most of us learned the alphabet at a young age, perhaps by singing the ABC song. But do you think you could say the alphabet backward starting with Z? Here's how the backward alphabet looks:

ZYXWVUTSRQPONMLKJIHGFEDCBA

This is easier to learn if you employ a technique called *chunking*, where you break the sequence of letters into easier-to-remember chunks:

ZYXWV UTSRQ **PONML** KJIHG FEDCBA

After a few days of practice, you should be able to whiz through it and amaze your friends.

If the alphabet is a bit too daunting, try spelling your name (first and last) or your city and state backward. This task requires concentration and some visualization. It's also a great brain exercise to do while stopped in traffic or waiting in line.

Day 6: Use your nondominant hand.

This a great kick-starter for a brain workout and one we frequently incorporate into our classes. Plus, it's easy to do (well, sort of). Simply switch your writing utensil from your dominant hand to your nondominant hand. So, if you're right-handed, put your pen in your left hand. Now sign your name, first and last, as if you were signing a check.

Not exactly effortless, is it? The opposite side of your brain is involved in a motor movement that it usually leaves alone. It's as if one side of your brain calls the other side and says, "Hey, you're in charge of writing today."

You can do this exercise with other tasks besides writing. For instance, try brushing your teeth with your nondominant hand. Watch out—that toothbrush might get frisky!

Day 7: Enhance your visual/perceptual memory.

Look at the following series of shapes for ten seconds:

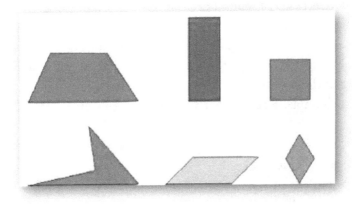

Now cover the shapes with a piece of paper (no cheating!). Redraw the figures in the following space as you saw them here:

How did you do?

Day 8: Practice spaced retrieval of memory.

Memorize this number: 82-1473.

Now, take your eyes away from the number and count backward from thirty by threes: 30, 27, 24, and so on.

Can you remember that number after the math exercise?

The ability to recall information after becoming distracted takes some effort and practice. This technique of memory rehearsal is called *spaced retrieval* and was developed in 1978 by Landauer and Bjork. The goal is to repeat the information back to yourself at increasingly longer intervals of time.

Start by repeating the number immediately, then wait for a minute before retrieving, then four or five minutes. Create a distraction (like the subtraction exercise) and then see if you can still recall the number, or substitute names or addresses instead of a number.

Day 9: Use the method of loci.

The method of Loci is a well-established technique that was known and used in ancient Greece. It involves the imaginary placement of items (like grocery or to-do lists) into various locations in an architectural structure, such as your own home or apartment. By creating a "memory palace," you can much more readily recall the items on the list.

As an example, let's say that we have the following items to purchase today:

- Loaf of bread
- Postage stamps
- Tennis balls
- Peanut butter
- Light bulbs

Now imagine that you are approaching your own home. As you pull into the driveway, you notice that you have rolled over something squishy with your car. When you get out and look under the car, you see that you have squashed a big, once-fluffy **loaf of bread**. Now approach your front door. As you do so, you notice that there is a letter stuck in your door frame covered with **stamps**. Go through your door and walk into your living room. Suddenly, you stumble, because the floor is covered with bright yellow **tennis balls.** Now proceed to the kitchen. You see that the kitchen sink is full of gooey, brown **peanut butter**. Over the sink is a single **light bulb** dangling from the ceiling.

Notice how it helps to paint a vivid picture and to involve the senses as much as possible. Although this scenario is a bit ridiculous, once you create it, you will find that it is difficult to forget the items.

Day 10: Practice a foreign language.

One of the best things you can do to keep your neurons flexible and communicative is to learn a foreign language. Even learning a few words will do. The reason? Forcing yourself to communicate in a different language pushes the brain out of its comfort zone, making it create new neural pathways. The same is true when learning to play a new piece of music when you play an instrument.

Our suggestion? Start small. Learn how to say "good morning," "please," and "thank you" in a new language every week. Rehearse the new words occasionally. See how long you can retain those phrases.

Day 11: Mix it up.

Have you ever driven somewhere and arrived at your destination only to wonder how you got there? Today's brain exercise involves doing something you do routinely, such as driving your car, and doing it differently, thus shutting off the "automatic pilot." The idea is to change your pattern so that your brain is forced to pay attention. Here are some ideas to get you going:

- If you are usually the driver when your family goes out, sit in the backseat and let somebody else drive.
- Take a completely different route to work, school, or the grocery store. Notice the different street names and landmarks of your new route.
- Tune the car radio to a different radio station—if you usually listen to country western, try classical or rock. If you prefer talk radio, try a music station.
- Try starting the car with your eyes closed, fishing out the correct key and inserting it into the ignition. (Now, please, *don't* drive with your eyes closed!)

Day 12: Interpret information upside down.

Though it may seem silly, a good brain stimulator is simply turning something (a picture, photo, written text) upside down and then trying to interpret it. You can start with whatever you have available, such as family photos, book covers, or artwork. Flip the object, and see what your brain makes of it. You may be surprised at how differently you perceive things when reversed.

Day 13: Play the "ten things" game.

This is a fun game for a group or a family, but you can also play alone. Take an ordinary object and then come up with ten different "things" for which the object might be used. For example, a pencil might be a baton, an arrow, a drum stick, a dental instrument, a stirring utensil, or a nail file. See how quickly you can come up with the ten items.

Day 14: Learn Sudoku.

Sudoku is a logic-based, number-placement puzzle. The objective is to fill a 9×9 grid with digits so that each column, each row, and each of the nine 3×3 subgrids that compose the grid contains all of the digits from 1 to 9. The puzzle comes with a few of the boxes already filled in.[52] Here is an example using a 3x3 grid:

	2	4	
1			3
4			2
	1	3	

Day 15: Practice Mathdoku.

Mathdoku puzzles are similar in some respects to Sudoku puzzles in that they take the form of a grid of numbers with blank squares to be filled in based on logical reasoning. Unlike Sudoku, however, Mathdoku relies on mathematics to solve the

---

52 "Sodoku," Wikipedia, Last Modified June 1, 2016, https://en.wikipedia.org/wiki/Sudoku.

puzzle. As in Sudoku, the goal of each puzzle is to fill a grid with digits—1 through 4 for a 4×4 grid, 1 through 5 for a 5×5, and so on—so that no digit appears more than once in any row or column. Grids range in size from 3×3 to 9×9. In addition, Mathdoku grids are divided into heavily outlined groups of cells called *cages*, and the numbers in the cells of each cage must produce a certain "target" number when combined using a specified mathematical operation (either addition, subtraction, multiplication, or division). Mathdoku puzzles go by several names, such as KenKen,[53] and can be found in the games section of many newspapers.

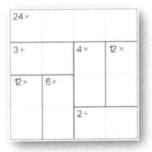

Day 16: Use a new word each day.

Purchase a word-a-day calendar and try to use the new word several times during the day.

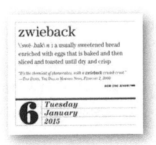

Day 17: Go to a museum.

Go to a museum or an art gallery and read the informational cards at each exhibit.

---

53 "KenKen," Wikipedia, Last Modified May 26, 2016, https://en.wikipedia.org/wiki/KenKen.

Day 18: Learn to juggle.

Learn to juggle three objects. A great way to do this is by purchasing the book *Juggling for the Complete Klutz*.[54] The book comes with three small beanbags, which are much easier to catch than hard balls.

Day 19: Listen to music.

Listening to music is very neurobic. If you have cable TV, you likely have several music channels available. Better yet, if you attend a live performance, you're combining both neurobics and socialization. Hint: try listening to a genre of music different from your usual favorite. For instance, if you normally listen to country western music, try listening to some classical music.

Day 20: Learn tai chi.

Tai chi, the ancient Chinese martial arts practice, provides many health and stress-reducing benefits. The best way to learn tai chi is by taking a class; however, you can also view an instructional DVD.

Day 21: Sense your environment.

Sit in a chair, close your eyes, and simply listen to the environment that surrounds you. Try to identify the sounds you hear and the aromas you smell. Sense the feeling of the air on your skin. This exercise is especially neurobic if you do it outdoors.

---

54 John Cassidy and B. C. Rimbeaux, *Juggling for the Complete Klutz*, 4th ed. (Palo Alto, CA: Klutz Press, 1994).

Day 22: Initiate a social interaction.

We spend a lot of time in public settings without interacting with the people around us. Try initiating a short conversation with someone in a waiting room or while in line at the supermarket.

Day 23: Learn a poem.

Pick a favorite poem and read it out loud. Keep practicing on a daily basis until you can recite it from memory.

Day 24: Learn to cook an ethnic dish.

Pick an ethnic cuisine outside your usual culinary repertoire. Research a recipe and try preparing it. The Internet is a great place to find recipes, and YouTube has thousands of short instructional videos on preparing ethnic dishes.

Day 25: Construct words with a word finder.

Use the following letters to construct words with at least three or more letters:

A E L S K

You get extra credit if you use all five letters. The solution can be found in appendix 6.

Day 26: Take a hike.

Take a hike in a park. Taking a walk in a natural setting activates many areas of the brain. See how many different types of flora and fauna you can identify. Close your eyes and take note of the sounds around you. Touch the different textures of tree bark. Smell the air, and feel the wind and sun on your skin.

Day 27: Grow a plant.

If you don't have a garden, but you do have a sunny window, plant an indoor herb garden. Fresh thyme and oregano are great herbs to have on hand for cooking. They are also quite aromatic.

Day 28: Learn your dry cleaners' names.

Choose a shop you frequent, such as your dry cleaners, and learn the names of the people who work there. Use mnemonic tags to help you remember their names. For example: Silly Sara, Raggedy Ralph, Too Tall Tina, and so on. The sillier the association, the more likely you are to remember their names. Greet them by name when you drop off or pick up your laundry.

Day 29: Assemble a jigsaw puzzle.

Choose an appealing image, and set up a card table somewhere where it can be left undisturbed for several days. Take breaks during your normal daily routine to fit a few pieces together. When you've completed the puzzle, consider donating it to a senior center or retirement community.

Day 30: Create a memory palace.

Memorize your grocery list by creating a "memory palace." See appendix 5 for an example of how to create a memory palace.

Day 31: Color.

Remember how much fun it was when you were a kid to get out your box of crayons and color a page from a coloring book? Well, coloring is not just for kids. Did you know that coloring activates many different parts of your brain? And adult coloring books are big sellers these days. You can find thousands of adult coloring pages online. Try it, and you will find that coloring is great for all ages.

Appendix 5: The Memory Palace

A *MEMORY PALACE* IS a mnemonic device to aid in placing information into and retrieving it from long-term memory. This technique is also referred to as the *method of loci*. Loci means "places" in Greek.

This technique uses imagery to aid memory. Images are often easier to recall than words. How many times have you thought to yourself, "I can't remember her name, but I can see her face in my memory"? The technique is attributed to the Greek poet Simonides (c.556–c.468 BCE). According to a legend passed on by the Roman statesman Cicero, the technique was discovered at a banquet in Thessaly that Simonides attended in order to present a lyric poem written in praise of the host. Simonides was called outside shortly after his performance, and, during his absence, the roof of the banqueting hall suddenly collapsed, crushing the other diners and mangling many of their corpses beyond recognition. Simonides, however, found he was able to identify the bodies (important for proper burial) by consulting his visual memory image of the people sitting around the banquet table, which enabled him to identify the corpses according to where they were found.[55]

As an example, let's create a memory palace to memorize a shopping list. Here's a hypothetical shopping list:

1. Bananas
2. Onions
3. Cottage cheese

---

55 "Ancient Imagery Mnemonics," Nigel J. T. Thomas, Stanford Encyclopedia of Philosophy, 2014, http://plato.stanford.edu/entries/mental-imagery/ancient-imagery-mnemonics.html.

4. Clothespins
5. Bottled water
6. Laundry detergent
7. Peanut butter
8. Light bulb
9. AA batteries

When given a list of items to memorize, on average, most individuals can recall about seven items.[56] We'll try for nine.

Cover up the list, and see how many items you can recall.

Now let's build a memory palace. Imagine that you are approaching your driveway in your car. You park your car and step out onto the driveway. You take a few steps when, all of sudden, you slip and fall. You notice that someone has left a **banana** peel on the ground. "Huh," you think to yourself. "How careless."

You pick yourself up, and it suddenly starts raining onions. You cover your head from the falling **onions** and run to the front door, where you are surprised to see a child's swimming pool filled to the brim with **cottage cheese**. And, even more interesting, there is a famous movie star sitting in the cottage cheese (pick one of your favorite stars). "How odd," you think.

Next, you fish out your house keys and unlock the front door. Upon entering your house, you immediately notice a military-style formation of animated **clothespins** marching back and forth at your feet. "Now that's certainly strange," you mutter to yourself.

You step over the marching clothespins and enter your living room, where you see six **bottles of water** dancing on the sofa. "Hmm. Dancing water bottles. What's next?" you think to yourself.

A you head for the kitchen, you pass by the dining table on which sits a huge, bright orange box of Tide **laundry detergent**. The box is so bright that you have to shield your eyes against the glare. "Gosh, that's bright!" you exclaim.

---

56 Lauren Schenkman, "In the Brain, Seven Is a Magic Number," *ABC News*, December 6, 2009, http://abcnews.go.com/Technology/brain-memory-magic-number/story?id=9189664.

In the kitchen, you stare in amazement at the sink. It's completely full of **peanut butter**. You stick a finger in the gooey mess and take a taste. "Yup, that's good peanut butter," you comment. Over the sink hangs a bare **light bulb** swinging on a long cord. You notice your shadow swaying as the light bulb swings back and forth.

Suddenly your cell phone chimes. You take the phone from your pocket and see that the screen displays a message: **AA batteries!**

Now you've created a memory palace with nine stops, each representing an item on your shopping list. Mentally go through your memory palace several times. Then write down the nine items on your list. Did you get them all? See how simple it is to create large memory palaces using different rooms and items in your home? You'll be amazed by the lengthy list you'll be able to memorize.

Appendix 6: Word Scramble Solutions

SOLUTION TO **Day 25: Construct words with a word finder** from appendix 4.

AELSK

1. Ale	10. Lea
2. Ales	11. Leak
3. Ask	12. <u>Leaks</u>
4. Elk	13. Sake
5. Elks	14. Sale
6. Kale	15. Sea
7. <u>Kales</u>	16. Seal
8. Lake	17. <u>Slakes</u>
9. <u>Lakes</u>	

Underlined words get extra points for using all five letters.

Appendix 7: Sample Progress Chart

	Mon	Tue	Wed	Thu	Fri	Sat	Sun	Weekly totals
Physical exercise								
Nutrition								
Neurobics								
Socialization								
Stress management								
Daily totals								

Each day, assess how you did on each pillar. If you feel that you did a great job, give yourself 5 points; so-so, give yourself 3 points; not so well, 1 point. Total each day, then, at the end of the week, calculate the weekly totals. Score yourself as follows:

140–175	Great job!
105–139	You're getting there.
70–104	Try a little harder.
35–69	Better luck next week.

Bibliography

Alzheimer's Association. "2015 Alzheimer's Disease Facts and Figures." *Alzheimer's & Dementia* 11, no. 3 (2015): 332–416.

Barnes, Deborah E., and Kristine Yaffe. "The Projected Effect of Risk Factor Reduction on Alzheimer's Disease Prevalence." *The Lancet Neurology* 10, no. 9 (2011): 819–28. doi:10.1016/S1474-4422(11)70072-2.

Birdsall, Timothy C. "5-Hydroxytroptophan: A Clinically-Effective Serotonin Precursor." *Alternative Medicine Review* 3, no. 4 (1998): 271–80.

Burrow, Marian. "Eating Well." *The New York Times,* March 29, 1995. http://www.nytimes.com/1989/11/15/garden/eating-well-marian-burros.html.

Carter, Rita. *The Human Brain Book.* New York: DK, 2009.

Carter, Sherrie Bourg. "Has Sleep and Stress Become a Vicious Cycle in Your Life? Why Sleep Should Be on the Top of Your To-Do List." *Psychology Today,* May 27, 2011. https://www.psychologytoday.com/blog/high-octane-women/201105/has-sleep-and-stress-become-vicious-cycle-in-your-life.

Cassidy, John, and B. C. Rimbeaux. *Juggling for the Complete Klutz.* 4th ed. Palo Alto, CA: Klutz Press, 1994.

Chang, Chia-Yu, Der-Shin Ke, and Jen-Yin Chen. "Essential Fatty Acids and Human Brain." *Acta Neurologica Taiwanica* 18, no. 4 (2009): 231–41.

Cherniack, E. Paul, Bruce R. Troen, Hermes J. Florez, Bernard A. Roos, and Silvina Levis. "Some New Food for Thought: The Role of Vitamin D in the Mental Health of Older Adults." *Current Psychiatry Reports* 11, no. 12 (2009): 12–19.

Cherniack, E. Paul, Hermes Florez, Bernard A. Roos, Bruce R. Troen, and Silvina Levis. "Hypovitaminosis D in the Elderly: From Bone to Brain." *The Journal of Nutrition Health and Aging* 12, no. 6 (2008): 366–73.

Conquer, Julie A., Mary C. Tierney, Julie Zecevic, William J. Bettger, and Rory H. Fisher. "Fatty Acid Analysis of Blood Plasma of Patients with Alzheimer's Disease, Other Types of Dementia, and Cognitive Impairment." *Lipids* 35, no. 12 (2000): 1305–12.

Davidson, Richard J., with Sharon Begley. *The Emotional Life of Your Brain: How Its Unique Patters Affect the Way You Think, Feel, and Live—and How You Can Change Them.* New York: Plume, 2013.

De la Monte, Suzanne M., and Jack R. Wands. "Alzheimer's Disease Is Type 3 Diabetes—Evidence Reviewed." *Journal of Diabetes Science and Technology* 2, no. 6 (2008): 1101–13.

Devi, Gayatri. *A Calm Brain: Unlocking Your Natural Relaxation System.* New York: Penguin, 2012.

Dharmarajan, T. S., G. U. Adiga, and Edward P. Norkus. "Vitamin B12 Deficiency. Recognizing Subtle Symptoms in Older Adults." *Geriatrics* 58, no. 3 (2003): 37–8.

Diament, Michelle. "How Friendship Keeps Our Brains Healthy." *Life Reimagined,* May 21, 2015. https://lifereimagined.aarp.org/stories/37251--How-Friendship-Keeps-Our-Brains-Healthy?cmp=SN-TWTTR-LR-POST-2015&sf38363302=1.

Dimpfel, Wilfried, A. Kler, E. Kriesl, and Ingrid Katharina Keplinger-Dimpfel. "Source Density Analysis of the Human EEG after Ingestion of a Drink Containing Decaffeinated Extract of Green Tea Enriched with L-Theanine and Theogallin." *Nutritional Neuroscience* 10, nos. 3–4 (2007): 169–80. doi:10.1080/03093640701580610.

Doidge, Norman. *The Brain that Changes Itself: Stories of Personal Triumph from the Frontiers of Brain Science.* New York: Penguin Books, 2007.

Duhigg, Charles. *The Power of Habit: Why We Do What We Do in Life and Business.* New York: Random House, 2012.

Eagleman, David. *Incognito: The Secret Lives of the Brain.* New York: Pantheon Books, 2011.

Fernandez, Alvaro, and Elkhonon Goldberg, with Pascale Michelon. *The SharpBrains Guide to Brain Fitness: How to Optimize Brain Health and Performance at Any Age.* San Francisco: SharpBrains, 2013.

Foer, Joshua. *Moonwalking with Einstein: The Art and Science of Remembering Everything.* New York: Penguin Press, 2011.

Gediman, Corinne L., with Francis M. Crinella. *Brainfit: 10 Minutes a Day for a Sharper Mind and Memory.* Nashville: Rutledge Hill Press, 2005.

Gutkencht, Lise, Christian Jacob, Alexander Strobel, Claudia Kriegebaum, Johannes Muller, Yong Zeng, Christoph Markert, Andrea Escher, Jens Wendland, Andreas Reif, Rainald Mossner, Cornelius Gross, Burkhard Brocke, and Klaus-Peter Lesch. "Tryptophan Hydroxylase-2 Gene Variation Influences Personality Traits and Disorders Related to Emotional Dysregulation." *The International Journal of Neuropsychopharmacology* 10, no. 3 (2007): 309–20.

Hartshorn, Joshua K., and Laura T. Germine. "When Does Cognitive Function Peak? The Asynchronous Rise and Fall of Different Cognitive Abilities Across the Life Span." *Psychological Science* 26, no. 4 (2015): 433–43. doi:10.1177/0956797614567339.

Hillman, Charles H., Kirk I. Erickson, and Arthur F. Kramer. "Be Smart, Exercise Your Heart: Exercise Effects on Brain and Cognition." *Nature Reviews Neuroscience* 9, no. 1 (2008): 58–65. doi:10.1038/nrn2298.

Honea, Robyn A., Eric D. Vidoni, Russell H. Swerdlow, and Jeffrey M. Burns. "Maternal Family History Is Associated with Alzheimer's Disease Biomarkers." *Journal of Alzheimer's Disease* 31, no. 3 (2012): 659–68. doi:10.3233/JAD-2012-120676.

Horrocks, Lloyd A., and Young K. Yeo. "Health Benefits of Docosahexaenoic Acid (DHA)." *Pharmacological Research* 40, no. 3 (1999): 211–25. doi:10.1006/phrs.1999.0495.

Kahnman, Daniel. *Thinking, Fast and Slow.* New York: Farrar, Straus and Giroux, 2011.

Kalmijn, S., Edith Feskens, L. J. Launer, and D. Kromhout. "Polyunsaturated Fatty Acids, Antioxidants, and Cognitive Function in Very Old Men." *American Journal of Epidemiology* 145, no. 1 (1996): 33–41. doi:10.1093/oxfordjournals.aje.a009029.

Kaplan, Jay R., Stephen Manuck, Thomas B. Clarkson, F. M. Lusso, and D. M. Taub. "Social Status, Environment and Atherosclerosis in Cynomolgus Monkeys." *Arteriosclerosis* 2, no. 5 (1982): 359–68. doi:10.1161/01. ATV.2.5.359.

Katz, Lawrence C., and Manning Rubin. *Keep Your Brain Alive: 83 Neurobic Exercises to Help Prevent Memory Loss & Increase Mental Fitness.* New York: Workman, 2014.

Kiraly, Stephen J., Michael A. Kiraly, Rick D. Hawe, and Naila Makhani. "Vitamin D as a Neuroactive Substance: Review." *Scientific World Journal* 26, no. 6 (2006): 125–39. doi:10.1100/tsw.2006.25.

Kirby, Elizabeth D., Aaron Friedman, D. Covarrubias, C. Ying, W. G. Sun, K. A. Goosens, R. M. Sapolsky, and D. Kaufer. "Basolateral Amygdala

Regulation of Adult Hippocampal Neurogenesis and Fear-Related Activation of Newborn Neurons." *Molecular Psychiatry* 17, no. 5 (2012): 527–36. doi:10.1038/mp.2011.71.

Kurzweil, Ray. *How to Create a Mind: The Secret of Human Thought Revealed.* New York: Viking, 2012.

Leiva, Jorge Garcia, Julio Martinez Salgado, Jose Estradas, Aldo Torre, and Misael Uribe. "Pathophysiology of Ascites and Dilutional Hyponatremia: Contemporary Use of Aquaretic Agents." *Annals of Hepatology* 6, no. 4 (2007): 214–21.

Mandal, Ananya. "Hippocampus Functions." *News Medical,* January 14, 2014. http://www.news-medical.net/health/Hippocampus-Functions.aspx.

Maslanka, Chris, and David Owen. *Neurobics: Create Your Own Brain Training Program.* New York: Reader's Digest, 2010.

Medina, John J. *Brain Rules: 12 Principles for Surviving and Thriving at Work, Home, and School.* Seattle: Pear Press, 2008.

Ramachandran, V. S. *The Tell-Tale Brain: A Neuroscientist's Quest for What Makes Us Human.* New York: W. W. Norton, 2011.

Ratey, John J., with Eric Hagerman. *Spark: The Revolutionary New Science of Exercise and the Brain.* New York: Little, Brown, 2008.

Robinson, Jo. *Eating on the Wild Side: The Missing Link to Optimum Health.* New York: Little, Brown, 2013.

Sapolsky, Robert M. *Why Zebras Don't Get Ulcers* (3rd ed.). New York: Henry Holt, 2004.

Schenkman, Lauren. "In the Brain, Seven Is a Magic Number." *ABC News,* December 6, 2009. http://abcnews.go.com/Technology/brain-memory-magic-number/story?id=9189664.

Singh, Narendra, Mohit Bhalla, Prashanti de Jager, and Marilena Gilca. "An Overview on Ashwagandha: A Rasayana (Rejuvenator) of Ayurveda." *African Journal of Traditional, Complementary and Alternative Medicines* 8 (2011): 208–13. doi:10.4314/ajtcam.v8i5S.9.

Szalavitz, Maia. "Social Isolation, Not Just Feeling Lonely, May Shorten Lives." *Time,* March 26, 2013. http://healthland.time.com/2013/03/26/social-isolation-not-just-feeling-lonely-may-shorten-lives/.

Talbot, Shawn. *The Cortisol Connection: Why Stress Makes You Fat and Ruins Your Health—and What You Can Do About It.* Alameda, CA: Hunter House, 2002.

Von Der Heide, Rebecca, Govinda Vyas, and Ingrid R. Olson. "The Social Network-Network: Size Is Predicted by Brain Structure and Function in the Amygdala and Paralimbic Regions." *Social Cognitive and Affective Neuroscience* 9, no. 12 (2014): 1962–72.

Warner, Melanie. *Pandora's Lunchbox: How Processed Food Took Over the American Meal.* New York: Scribner, 2013.

Winter, Bernward, Caterina Breitenstein, Frank C. Mooren, Klaus Voelker, Manfred Fobkes, Anja Lechtermann, Karsten Krueger, Albert Fromme, Catharina Korsukewitz, Agnes Floel, and Stefan Knecht. "High Impact Running Improves Learning." *Neurobiology of Learning and Memory* 87, no. 4 (2007): 597–609. doi:10.1016/j.nlm.2006.11.003.

Yang, Quanhe, Zefeng Zhang, Edward W. Gregg, W. Dana Flanders, Robert Merritt, and Frank B. Hu. "Added Sugar Intake and Cardiovascular Disease Mortality Among US Adults." *JAMA Internal Medicine* 174, no. 4 (2014): 516–24. doi:10.1001/jamainternmed.2013.13563.

About the Authors

MEREDITH PATTERSON, RN, BSN, CRRN is co-owner of Brainstorm Mind Fitness, a company whose mission is to educate the public on strategies to keep your brain healthy as you age, improve cognitive functions, and reduce the likelihood of developing Alzheimer's disease.

PETE GOODWIN is co-owner of Brainstorm Mind Fitness, along with Meredith Patterson. Prior to founding Brainstorm Mind Fitness, Pete managed memory-care facilities in south central Texas and was administrator of an in-home senior care business. Pete is a graduate of the Ohio State University and served as a US Army medical corpsman in Vietnam in the early 1970s.

CPSIA information can be obtained
at www.ICGtesting.com
Printed in the USA
LVHW080009260219
608759LV00008B/296/P